ANCIENT YOGA

FOR MODERN PRACTITIONERS

FIVE-MINUTE PRACTICES FOR INNER PEACE

by

LEILA WORBY

FROM THE TINY ACORN . . .
GROWS THE MIGHTY OAK

www.acornpublishingllc.com
For information, address:
Acorn Publishing, LLC
3943 Irvine Blvd. Ste. 218
Irvine, CA 92602

Ancient Yoga for Modern Practitioners: Five-Minute Practices for Inner Peace
Copyright © 2021 Leila Worby

Cover design by Damonza.com
Interior design and formatting by Debra Cranfield Kennedy and Lacey Impellizeri-Papenhausen

Printed in the United States of America

ISBN-13: 978-1-952112-85-0 (hardcover)
ISBN-13: 978-1-952112-84-3 (paperback)

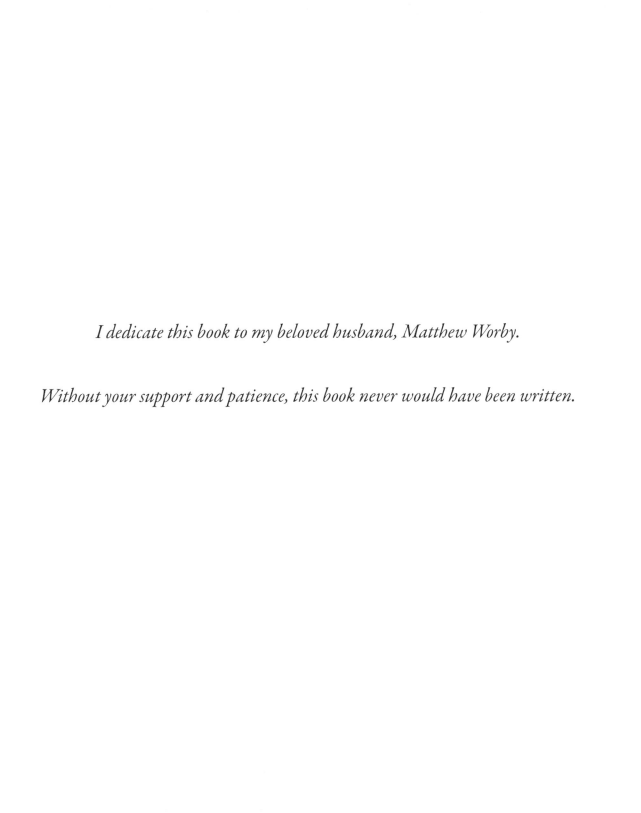

I dedicate this book to my beloved husband, Matthew Worby.

Without your support and patience, this book never would have been written.

TABLE OF CONTENTS

INTRODUCTION

For over a decade, I have practiced and taught *yoga* and witnessed its profound effects. I decided to write this book to help others achieve a balanced approach to life. I believe anyone new to the path of *yoga* can benefit from a personalized transformational *yoga* practice that extends beyond basic knowledge of the poses and includes information about why certain techniques are used. This book offers techniques for people who struggle because of negative self-talk, burn-out, depression, anxiety, and panic attacks while trying to keep up with the demands of modern society.

When stress impacts the nervous system, it affects how the body, mind, and emotions function. This book explains how *yoga* can bring the nervous system back into harmony and how *you* can craft a *yoga* practice that will bring your unique body back into balance.

This book explores *pranayama* (breathing techniques), *mantras* (sound), *mudras* (hand gestures), *namaskars* (movement meditations or salutations), and *asana* (poses). The practices are broken down into five-minute sessions for the meditative practices and fifteen-minute sessions for the movement meditations, allowing you to customize your practice according to the duration and the style of practice that fits into your life at any given moment.

Yoga is all about living in flow with nature, and this book will provide you with techniques to do just that.

CHAPTER 1

The Body's Systems

HOW MODERN SOCIETY AFFECTS STRESS LEVELS

As a species, we haven't developed much physiologically beyond the caveman's level. Human physiology has evolved and adapted to accommodate its current surroundings but not to a point that can fully accommodate modern technology. Right now, most of us live in a world that requires us to be continuously connected to our screens, operating chiefly in manmade environments lit up by artificial lighting. Some of us spend a lot of time in our cars or other vehicles. The constant connection to our phones and screens directs our attention externally—all the time. Previous generations had the benefit of mindfully being in the moment in deep communion with the elements of nature and with loved ones. This screen-free mode allowed the brain to naturally and organically unwind and to start fresh again with renewed energy. Today, it remains challenging for people to experience a natural shift between brainwaves for optimal well-being. The frequency of your brainwaves changes constantly over the course of your day, depending on which stimuli trigger your nervous system. We tend to produce a brainwave environment that is caused by stress and the Sympathetic Nervous System (the SNS will be explained in greater detail further on.) This environment can be characterized by increased beta waves (in high frequencies responsible for agitation and anxiousness), decreased alpha waves (responsible for relaxation, focus and flow), and sometimes low delta waves (responsible for deep sleep) and theta waves (responsible for a state of deeper relaxation than alpha, the place just before we fall asleep or just as we wake up).

We have successfully removed the critical elements of well-being and function and replaced them with our technology-centered environments. If we do not develop tools to be mindful and direct our attention internally again, stress, exhaustion, burn-out, and depression will inevitably follow.

A friend of mine who performs neurotherapy generated a brain map that measured my brainwaves. We are both avid meditators, and we were excited to see how we could actually measure my shift into a state dominated by alpha brain waves when I practiced one of the *kriyas* or five-minute meditations that will later be outlined in this book. Alpha brainwaves are associated with mediation and a sense of calm and peacefulness and with focus and creative flow. There is a direct correlation between raising alpha brainwaves and a reduction in feeling anxious. Since stress is the main culprit when it comes to producing unfavorable brainwaves, we need to understand just how it manifests.

COMMON SYMPTOMS AND LONG-TERM CONSEQUENCES OF STRESS

When our nervous system is under stress, it can initially manifest as acne, hair loss, rashes, digestive problems, headaches, and sleep disturbances. We may also suffer from weight changes, high blood pressure, chest pain, and heart palpitations. In our twenties and thirties, and sometimes, much earlier, these symptoms usually start appearing. If we don't do something about them, they can have lethal effects in our forties and fifties.

Many people struggle to cope with life pressures, such as managing a career and family life, while maintaining a sense of purpose and well-being. Heart disease, stroke, and other cardiovascular diseases are common more mature symptoms of stress. There is a strong association between chronic stress and depression. Stress can cause anxiety and panic attacks. The body has learned to respond to stress by getting more and more anxious, which sometimes culminates in a panic attack. Stress also takes a toll on your reproductive abilities. It's useful to be in a state of relaxation and receptivity when you are trying to conceive.

The earlier you start combatting the signs of stress, the easier it is to return to balance. The longer you let the stress shift you away from equilibrium, the harder it is to restore it. The good news is that it's never too late to make a change. In as few as thirty days you can ditch a bad habit or create a good one.

BALANCING THE NERVOUS SYSTEM WITH *YOGA*

When we get stressed, our Sympathetic Nervous System (SNS) is overstimulated. The SNS prompts the fright-flight response in our reptilian brains. This part of our nervous system gets triggered when we feel stressed or threatened or when too much of our attention is directed externally. When our attention is directed externally our senses are used to process information outside of ourselves. Internal attention on the other hand has to do with our imagination, planning and ultimately our creativity and independent thought process. When the SNS governs us, we are unable to effectively listen to other people or tap into our own creativity. We are running a hundred miles per hour with blinders on. This chaotic mode depletes our energy and senses.

Yoga provides a toolset that can be implemented to balance our nervous system and even stimulate the Parasympathetic Nervous System (PNS). When the PNS gets triggered, it prompts us to rest and digest. Activating this part of our nervous system enables us to listen and digest information, slowing us down enough to operate analytically and judiciously. By stimulating the PNS, we slow down our heart rate and decrease cortisol, the stress hormones, in our system.

We want to spend the majority of our productive time in a state that promotes focus and creativity. We want to achieve the state of flow where creative ideas spontaneously appear from the depths of our unconscious mind. And we can only enter that eureka state from a state of relaxation. There is a way to stimulate your nervous system to enter that state of relaxation, delay aging and promote mental and physical well-being: *yoga*.

MASTERING THE NERVOUS SYSTEM WITH THE BREATH

Yoga, initially, through the breath, can help stimulate the nervous system toward balance. Even three minutes of smooth, mindful, deep breathing without the addition of more refined or sophisticated *yogic* breathing techniques, improves attention, relaxation, and the ability to cope with a challenging situation.

To simplify meditation techniques, if you have a problem with focusing your attention, spend a couple of minutes mindfully observing your breath without interference. But if you are in severe emotional discord—depressed, anxious, stressed out, or about to have a panic attack—you need to manipulate your breath to make a more immediate shift. This is where *yogic* breathing techniques, also known as *pranayama*, can have a more profound effect than mindfulness as a stand-alone technique.

Pranayama is an incredibly efficient tool to manipulate your nervous system and, if practiced incorrectly, can cause both mental and physical harm. In fact, *yoga* initially received attention in the west because *Krishnamacharya* was able to stop his heart at will by manipulating his nervous system, mainly through the practice of *pranayama*. (*Krishnamacharya* is usually referred to as the father of modern *yoga*. His disciples made *Yoga* famous in the west.) This should illustrate just how powerful these practices are. If you want to feel safe when using the methods that will later be outlined in this book, go over them in person with a senior *yoga* teacher to ensure that you are executing them correctly.

One of *yoga's* foundational practices is the ability to direct attention inward at will. We call this *pratyahara*. We cultivate this state through breathing techniques and specific poses, and it must be practiced for years before one is prepared to enter deeper states of meditation. *Pratyahara* is the prerequisite to move on to the next level, which allows us to focus our attention, which is called *dharana*. It can be used to enter deeper states of meditation or to achieve optimal productivity. The beauty of learning these techniques is that you can choose to use your attention to be productive in the workplace or to shut down, rest, and restore.

I work with so many brilliant people that have the ability to hyper-focus their minds, but they can't shut them off. You must be the master of your mind. Your well-being relies on you having the tools to control your mind, even to a minimal degree.

So many people today cannot find the *off* button. The "rat race" leaves them feeling empty and without a sense of purpose. I have often encountered people who seem like the most successful individuals in Silicon Valley, but often, these people are in a state of deep depression. Why is this? Because, we are divine spiritual beings having a human, embodied, and materialistic experience.

The greatest misunderstanding of our kind, is that we have to "become" something and that we have to accumulate wealth in order to fill our inner void. Most societies reinforce these views, so very few of us manage to live in the moment without striving. We end up wasting our short time on this earth by chasing desires that, when consummated, only leave us feeling more empty than before. We can accumulate what we believe to be the ideal life or the perfect career or a garage full of luxury cars, only to feel that void greater than ever. Because the chase has ended, we got what we wanted, but we are still not fulfilled. At least as long as you're chasing, you are occupied. But for the "lucky" few who get there, the void becomes unbearable. Or rather the lack of knowledge of how to fill that void. The emptiness that you feel inside you, that can sometimes threaten to engulf you, wants to be filled with life force, not material objects.

INTEGRATING *YOGIC* TECHNIQUES IN YOUR LIFE FOR OPTIMAL RESULT

We are a function of our habits. A small but sustained change in practices can have great cumulative effects. It's better to do five minutes of *yoga* a couple times a day than it is to do an hour of *yoga* a couple times a month. You want to train your brain to enter the state of flow and stay there throughout the day. And when it strays, gently guide it back to your desired brainwave frequency. The best way of doing that is by using micro-meditations, also called *kriyas* (specific sets of exercises, breathing techniques, visualizations and sound *mantras* that unlock energy channels in the body). *Kriyas* focus your mind and shift your breathing patterns. Breath is the harness that commands the mind. Breath reels the mind in and directs it inward. You can choose where to go from there. For *yoga* beginners, the key is the breath.

I first discovered the effect of micro-meditations during a time when I had a very dedicated Ashtanga practice. I would rise before sunrise, drive to the *shala* (a space where *yoga* is shared and experienced) and complete a rigorous one-to two-hour practice every morning, six days a week. I would then go about my day observing how the steadiness of mind and level of relaxation, in essence, my *yoga* glow, would dissipate and vanish as my day progressed. I started to intuitively weave some of the *kriyas* I had learned from my meditation teachers into my day. I noticed how those techniques immediately pulled me back into a state of flow. I would do five minutes under a tree in a park after I dropped my youngest at kindergarten, five minutes before and after I taught my *yoga* classes, and five minutes before bedtime. This routine came to me intuitively. My being craved to be moved back into the state of flow throughout my entire day, not just during my physical *asana* practice that took place in the early morning hours. These micro-meditations became like small mind breaks for me and a crucial part of my well-being. The most important thing about them and all my *yoga* practice is that they are the highlights of my day. They are my sanctuary.

To use this system optimally it's useful to have an established practice of about twenty minutes a day to connect back to. To more effortlessly access the flow state, you first need to establish a familiarity with it. It's like filling up a pot with water. If it's already full, it's easier to make it overflow with just a few drops.

Yoga, as a complete system and way of life, works to promote your well-being by grounding you. It slows you down to a point where you can turn inward and tune into your true inner essence, which is part of the whole. By slowing down we are able to move beyond the chatter of mind and connect with our soul. This soul is just part of the greater soul or life force, that

Leila Worby

encompasses everything. Some people would refer to this life force as god or goddess.

As *yoga* practitioners, we also use nature to connect with the all-encompassing life force. Actual well-being relies on your ability to slow down and listen to your real needs, not your preprogrammed needs. This starts with your ability to connect with nature. Nature is just one, big macro-cosmos that plays a crucial part in balancing your micro-cosmos.

Connection to the flow of nature is particularly apparent to women. We can feel our bodies wax and wane with the moon phases, just like the tides ebb and flow with the pull of the moon. The connection between the human body and the water's ebbs and flows should make perfect sense. After all, we consist of about sixty percent water.

BUILDING A STRONG FOUNDATION

You can achieve a substantial foundational shift toward well-being without adding any *yogic* practices. Then, adding *yoga* will boost your inner fire, but the roof will fall in and destroy the house if the foundation isn't in order.

If you take anything away from this book, let it be the sentiment that you are a product of your daily habits. Shifting your patterns ever-so-slightly will have a massive impact on your well-being over time. Changing them significantly can be even more life-changing. Don't overlook small changes; they can create momentum for you to be able to make greater changes. But the key is to make changes that are sustainable in your life. When you are changing your behavior, do it gradually and slowly. You want to add a teaspoon of goodness and work your way toward a gallon.

Before adopting *yogic* practices that will change your life, you should ensure your sleep, your nutrition, your movement, and your relationships are in balance. Most *yogic* practices, apart from *pranayama*, are incredibly subtle. In order to fully benefit from and experience them, you need to attune yourself to your subtle body, also called your energy body. The movement from gross to subtle is a little like the difference between coffee and tea. Coffee is very much in your face, potent, and very tangible in its flavor and scent. Being attuned to your subtle body means tuning into the lighter, more complex flavors of tea. *Yoga* is a movement toward lightness in every choice of your day, and it starts with looking after your physical body.

SLEEP

Getting proper sleep is incredibly important when it comes to well-being. You burn fat when you sleep due to a hormonal secretion that only takes place in deep sleep. Don't deprive your body of that fine tuning by consuming too much caffeine or wine before you go to bed. Turn off screens an hour and a half before bedtime. Racing thoughts, or rumination, often leaves people sleepless. When I worked in a corporate environment, I suffered regularly from a replay of my entire day during the first half of my night. I then used the second half of the night to visualize and mentally prepare for all the emails and interactions I'd have the next day. This left me fuzzy-headed and slow to react the following day.

One good way of clearing your thoughts before bed is to journal about them. Put that to-do list on paper. That way, it's easier to let go of it. Or if it's a relationship that's got your mind turning all night, journal about how to improve it. Create a strategy, and consider solutions and deadlines in case improvement fails. Journaling is the cheapest form of therapy. It's a way to let your own inner guru solve your problems, which is the goal of most cognitive behavioral therapy, anyway. Also, journaling is more sleep-inducing than Netflix. If your mind is clear enough, you may love reading before bed. If you have time, take a long lavender bath and add some Epsom salts. Even taking a lukewarm shower can properly prepare you for your sleep journey. Guided meditation can also help you fall asleep. If you are still struggling to fall asleep, try the *yogic* techniques outlined later in this book. *Yoga* will help you clear your mind before sleep. or even during the day, should you need a reset.

FOOD

For many people, nutrition is the hardest habit to shift. Start by making a list of fruit and vegetables you enjoy. Then, fill your fridge with them, and try to eat them with every meal and as snacks when hungry between meals. A good strategy is to fill up on raw fruit and veggies before you have your main course. I eat a lot of Greek, Israeli, and Mexican food. I hate to cook, so I make it super simple: Greek salad; Israeli salad; and black bean, corn, and avocado salad. If I crave denser nutrition, I wrap the salad ingredients in a tortilla. I also like to eat a lot of almond butter on toast for density and protein. If your constitution craves meat, keep portions small, but try to eliminate it as much as you can. At the very least, choose organic and free-range meats.

There are hordes of vegan chefs sharing their latest and greatest recipes on social media. If you like to cook, let them inspire you. If you "fall off the wagon," please know there isn't a wagon to fall off of. Notice how you feel when you are eating whatever food you have deemed off-limits for yourself, and notice how your body feels afterward. Moving toward the right nutrition and a *yogic* way of eating means listening to your body and being present when you nourish your body. Do not eat in front of screens. Never beat yourself up because of food choices. Simply notice how they make you feel, and stick to your intention of eating healthy as much as you can. If you can eat healthy eighty percent of the time, you can "treat" yourself to a cheat meal once a week. After a while, you will only want to eat the foods that make your body feel light and happy. If you crave sweet stuff, turn toward honey and fruits—dates in particular.

Before you eat, take a moment to think about what had to happen to create the food in front of you—moon cycles, sun cycles, rain, farmers planting and harvesting, manufacturers processing, and drivers transporting. Visualize all of this before you eat. Then, become fully absorbed in the experience of eating. Make eating part of your meditation practice. You can even journal about the taste, texture, and smell of the food and how it makes you feel before and after you have ingested it.

As you go about your day, try to listen to your body, and notice your hunger when it is at its strongest. Make those times your meal times. My meal times fall during odd hours. I eat my main meals at 11 AM and 4 PM during the days when I don't have to be social. Discover when your body is actually hungry, and avoid eating just because the clock strikes a certain hour.

If you are struggling with hunger pangs between meals, try *prana mudra* (described in the mudra chapter of this book), which is often used to sustain people who are fasting for religious reasons because it provides an influx of life force that isn't derived from food.

DRINK

Getting enough water is essential to your well-being, but it's easy to overdo it and create an imbalance. Again, it is a question of honing the ability to turn inward and listen to what your body needs. Cultivate tapping into that quiet place by using the body as the instrument of your practice. Thirst can masquerade as hunger, so practice drinking water before you reach for a snack. But avoid drinking simply because you're bored. Adding cucumber and mint, or other natural flavors to water to tap into subtleness even more. In *yogic* philosophy, we are instructed to eat two to three times a day and never after sunset. When you eat, you should fill the stomach with fifty percent *sattvic* foods and twenty-five percent water and leave twenty-five percent space for the body to digest properly. Ice cold water is not recommended for optimal digestion; it's recommended only to drink lukewarm water. Again, it is best to stop ingesting stimulants such as coffee and alcohol after 5 PM and to limit your intake of these substances as much as you can.

OPTIMAL MOVEMENT AND USE OF THE SENSES

Avoid strenuous exercise because strenuous exercise, such as running and weight-lifting, triggers your hunger. Particularly if you're struggling with overeating, you want to avoid that trigger and instead, focus on a consistent, slow burn to target your fat layer.

In *yoga* we consider movement optimal if it doesn't make you perspire or lose your breath. In some traditions it's even taught to rub the sweat back into the skin if this happens, for hydration and life force maintenance. Ideally, you should flow from one pose to the next during your *yoga* practice with steadiness and ease. Again, we are looking for a smoothness of movement that works to soothe the nervous system. We are not looking for peaks and valleys as we manage our body through space. In fact, strenuous exercise is considered misguidance in *yoga* because it creates an imbalance in your energy levels. This is why I always recommend walking rather than running. It's more sustainable and less depleting over time.

Move for the joy of movement. Don't punish yourself. Think about the love you feel for the creature or human in your life that you love the most. Then extend that love and forgiveness to yourself.

To optimize our physical well-being we need to be careful with how we nourish and use our other senses. Simply exercising the body isn't enough, because the other senses trigger our nervous system which impacts the well-being of your physical body.

Nutrition is not only what we take in through our mouths but also what we take in through our eyes and ears. For optimal well-being, try to avoid violence, gore, drama and intrigue when you make your Netflix choice. Watch artistically beautiful shows that inspire creative urges in you. Make it a way of incorporating art into your life. Try to cut out anything that negatively affects your mood. To move myself into the state of flow in my everyday life I like to listen to *mantras* as a way of reconnecting to my practice. Music is a powerful tool with a big impact on your nervous system.

How we relate socially additionally has an impact on our nervous system and as such our physical well-being. The *yogic* scriptures urge you to stay away from gossip and feeble talk because they waste energy, depleting the physical and subtle bodies. You may have experienced that interacting with certain individuals leaves your feeling drained and negative. It's because engaging in drama and gossip guides your attention away from being grounded and resting in your center into all sorts of thought cycles that only feed the ego. If it is an intellectually stimulating conversation it might feed you, but as a general rule speech is considered the most crude form of communication in *yoga*, and it is when we are in flow with another human that true connection happens through our other senses.

CREATING A SOCIAL SUPPORT NETWORK

As a species, humans are flock animals. The tribe we surround ourselves with helps us confirm our own identity. The people in our lives work as mirrors that reflect our inner essence. Because of this interconnectedness, we must surround ourselves with positive people with whom we resonate. There are billions of people globally and plenty of opportunities to bring healthy relationships into your life. Don't stay in relationships that don't serve you. The older you get, the more you will realize time is of the essence. Choose your tribe wisely because they will either support you in moving toward your true inner essence or hold you back from it. If you haven't met your tribe and are feeling lonely, know this is normal from time to time throughout a lifetime. Dare to be on your own. In discomfort lies growth and eventually strength.

I went through a couple of moves to different countries before the availability of the internet. In the beginning I had a hard time meeting people, so I know the sadness and vulnerability loneliness can cause. My recommendation would be to search for a Meetup group with people who share your passions. For introverts, this can seem like an uncomfortable and nearly impossible task. However, discovering a social support network that allows you to be who you truly are is instrumental to your well-being. Challenge yourself to step outside of your comfort zone. Take classes that resonate with you. Practice making small talk. Finding just one good friend makes it worth the discomfort.

BALANCING CREATIVE ENDEAVORS AND WORKLOAD

When I became invested in *yoga*, I was juggling two baby boys who were seventeen months apart. Watching famous childless *yoga* practitioners sharing their extensive morning routines left me feeling like *yoga* wasn't for me. These social media influencers had the time to sample their tea, journal for hours, and practice *asana* (postural *yoga*) before strolling along the beach while smelling the morning sea breeze. It all felt so incredibly out of reach for someone in my situation. However, a consistent *yoga* practice is nothing like what's displayed on social media. In fact, the practice is like a flower. It starts off like a small investment of time, a seed that's planted and grows over time until it resembles a fully blossomed flower, all you need to do is water it regularly.

In *yoga*, the phases of a human life are divided into four stages. First, you're a student, learning about life and finding your path. This stage is all about you as an individual and your personal development. Second, you become a householder, focused on raising a family. This takes a great amount of energy because you must serve the people you brought into this world. A lot of self-reflection and growth is available during this chapter of your life. The transition can be rough as you understand your time is no longer your own. In the third stage, your practice and attention shift from your children to yourself as more time becomes available for deeper introspection. In a way, you become a forest dweller, one who retires in the woods in deep pursuit of your interests and spiritual duties. This is followed by the fourth stage, that of the *sannyasin*, one who renounces everything and lives a life of ascetics in preparation for the final passage. During ideal circumstances, living a rich life full of spirituality is possible throughout these stages. We don't need any special practices or circumstances to access the present moment. And this is the true *yoga*. But because most of us are imbalanced, the *yogic* techniques in this book are more relevant today than ever before. They can help you achieve balance. Over time these practices will become your sanctuary, your connection to the life force and pure love. Instead of searching externally for fulfillment, you will find it in your practice.

Regardless of what stage of life you are in, you must set aside time for physical well-being and time for creative endeavors, such as drawing, painting, writing, computer programming, or dancing. It is vital to tap into creativity daily, even for just a few minutes, to feel a sense of purpose and vitality and to enter the state of flow.

When you take time for yourself, you will have more to offer your children. When my kids were babies I made a point of taking a meditative walk with them in the stroller during their nap time. That was my way of taking care of my own physical being and accessing a meditative state at the same time. Eventually, my *yoga* practice took the place of my daily walk and is now my biggest outlet of my creativity. Find what resonates with you. It's essential to cultivate creativity to prevent burnout because when your inner fire dies, you won't have anything to give. If you put your own needs before your kids' needs, you will be fulfilled, and when your kids leave the nest, you will have interests of your own to enjoy. Make sure your children are safe and cared for, but make your own needs a priority.

MASTERING YOUR MIND

A balanced and stable emotional state is crucial for well-being. Usually our thought patterns or inner stories fuel strong emotions. The negative mind yaps on and on, and we believe the inner narrative, which is often filled with impatience, self-pity, and resentment. In some scriptures the pessimistic mind has been compared to a crazy monkey jumping from tree to tree.

To overcome this inhibiting state, it's useful to understand how the mind works, how to best relate to the mind, and how to digest strong emotions properly. The alternative is to allow less desirable, deep, repetitive thought patterns to form and reoccur.

In *yoga* we call these repetitive, ingrained thought patterns *samskaras*. *Samskaras* help the mind process information and make sense of surroundings. The samskaras become our behavioral patterns and are determined to a great extent by our environment and our genes. Our genes govern the nervous system and metabolism, and as such, they affect the brain's ability to produce and absorb neurotransmitters responsible for our emotional response. Our emotional response impacts the formation of our thoughts and whether they are positive or negative. You cannot change your genes or the traumas you have experienced. The only thing you have the power to do is to see your mind for what it is—limited and mostly toxic. If you observe its endless monologue, you can transcend it.

The Daoists believe that everyone is born into this world with different strengths of *qi* or life force. But even someone with a weak *qi* can build it and become even more powerful than people that were born with exceptionally strong *qi*, through consistent practice of the *Dao*. Essentially, *yogic* philosophy aligns with this belief and offers *yoga* as a way to overcome the negative mind by moving body and mind into stillness. In fact, *BKS Iyengar* overcame malaria, tuberculosis, typhoid fever, and general malnutrition through his dedicated *yoga* practice, and he became the most famous *yoga* master of modern times with a strong physical practice that he maintained into his nineties.

TRANSCENDENCE VERSUS EMBODIMENT— *YOGA* VERSUS *TANTRA*

There are a few steps to consider when you try to move beyond mind. The first is to slow down your thoughts to avoid knee-jerk reactions from becoming samskaras. When our mind is racing because our SNS is being continuously triggered, we tend to immediately adapt the simplistic "fight or flight response." The "fight or flight response" can become a negative, ingrained, and repetitive behaviour if we're not careful, that only works to create more stress in our lives. To access deeper more mature thought patterns and behaviours we need to slow down the activities of mind, so that we take time to pause, reflect and evaluate. We don't want our most primal impulses to become *Samskaras*. *Samskaras* are like deep grooves in a mountain side, created by the water flowing down from its top. Grooves that deepen and that eventually form the path for an entire river.

Accessing our most mature nature can be done by taking a few slow deep breaths. Slowing down helps you become a witness so you may observe the chatter of mind as a detached being. If you view your mind objectively from a witness standpoint, just as if you were watching a movie, you can respond less emotionally and calm its fluctuations. Once we slow down and calm the fluctuations of mind, we may eventually experience complete silence. And arrive at the final goal of *Classical Hatha Yoga*-unity with the life force, which you may call god or goddess.

In *Classical Hatha Yoga* it was advised to work towards experiencing this state in solitude, far away from the hustle and bustle of normal life, so that you wouldn't be distracted from your meditative practices. In addition the body was seen as something impure, something that was to be transcended. Often through the practice of austerities. Austerities are practices that refrain from worldly pleasures. They are characterized by denying bodily needs. Exemples are celibacy and poverty. And often in *yoga*—inner cleansing and meditation. They are practices of moving your attention away from your physical needs into the spiritual realm and ultimately transcend your physical body.

In *Tantra*, on the other hand, and this is really the main difference between the two paths, transcendence or going beyond the physical body into complete stillness, isn't the ultimate state. The ultimate state is the embodied state, when you use the body as a vehicle to liberation or unity with god. You experience this state when you move beyond being the witness and allow your consciousness to fully inhabit the body through the physical sensory experience at any given moment, without any judgment. It's a state of mindfully being in the present moment and reveling in pleasure and pain alike as you make every act a meditation.

My personal experience on the path of *yoga* powerfully illustrates the two paths. In my opinion, the *tantric* path is much more compelling and complete, particularly during the householder phase. Because it allows you to make every moment into *yoga*. The mundane everyday tasks and interactions that come with being a householder are the real *yoga*, not the fancy poses or the deep, mystical trance states. Real *yoga* happens in every interaction with other beings and when doing the dishes. Both paths have their merits. Ultimately the path one chooses depends on one's needs and preferences as well as what stage of life they're in. When you're at a junction of your life when solitude is available to you, transcendental practice might really resonate.

In the early days of getting deep into *yoga*, I was practicing for hours a day. I ate, breathed, and dreamed of *yoga*. I would do physical *yoga* and meditation for hours and then dream about doing advanced *yoga* poses that were not yet available or even known to me during the night. This living and dreaming *yoga* went on for years. It was as though I was supercharged with *yoga*. And as a result of my intense *yoga* practice, I started feeling very detached from my emotions and

Leila Worby

my social circle. I had no interest in the world of humans. All I wanted was the state that *yoga* took me to—a restful place of complete silence, stillness, emptiness, and soothing darkness that is known in *yogic* philosophy as *Shunya*, or *The Void*. Being an introvert, I enjoyed this detached state to such an extent that I didn't care to form deep relationships with my surroundings, outside of my immediate family. I was so mesmerized by this state that years passed before I was ready to move on from it. I am really grateful that I had my children as I went through this phase because they helped me stay grounded.

The void is like death, rest and stillness. And from *the void*, *spanda*, life force or vibration is born. Think of it like deep, restful sleep as compared to the state of being fully awake, acutely aware of the light, and vibrating with love. That really is the difference between the void and the *spanda*. When you're awake you enjoy experiencing the world like a child, through your senses. That experience of aliveness becomes the highest state, not the detached mystical trance that is also very enjoyable.

One of the reasons *the void* had such a pull on me was because it allowed me to not have to fully feel my emotions. They seemed simultaneously overwhelming and unimportant. Observing them from a detached third-person vantage point, and leaning on the teachings of reality being *Maya* or an illusion anyway, felt like a good and easy escape. I wasn't yet equipped with the tools to safely be present with my feelings and make that experience my practice. Being able to pause and observe your emotions from an objective viewpoint is the first step towards healing. To come full circle you must learn to not only calmly observe them, but how to fully be with them and eventually digest them. When we consider this as a movement of consciousness we find a movement from *the void* into *the spanda*. The void is necessary from time to time, because it allows us to pause, rest and reflect. But it's important not to get stuck there, regardless of how much we're enjoying the experience. Ideally the movement between these two states of consciousness is dynamic and changing as you move through life.

To move safely toward being present with your emotions, try bringing your attention from your head to what is known in *yogic* philosophy as the *hridaya*, the seat of the soul, that is located in your heart center. You relax into the center of your being (try visualizing your entire spine here and particularly the heart), and take a few deep breaths, to anchor your consciousness in the heart center.

Then lie down in a restorative pose, one that feels good to you—perhaps with your legs up the wall, or supported fish pose, my personal favorite (described and pictured under restorative poses). Enter the pose and breathe deeply for as many moments you need.

As you're ready, disconnect the emotion from the story attached to it. The story isn't real, and it's not essential. You may find it helpful to visualize the negative feeling you associate with the story. Does it have a color? A particular shape or temperature? Where does it seem to reside in the body? Does it move in a specific direction? Pull the emotion deep into the core of your being and feel it. Let it resonate in your physical body. Become one with it. Cry and howl as much as you want to until the sorrow or pain are gone. Let the emotion pass entirely through you. This is how to digest strong emotions. The big pitfall here is to start thinking of the story attached to the emotion. Then you're not digesting it. You must realize that the mind only sees a sliver of the truth, a sliver that is highly generalized. So in order to digest the emotion, do your best to focus on how it feels in your body and detach the story you're associating it with.

Often, we have been taught to eat something sweet to soothe pain, or to have a glass of wine to take the edge off, and that becomes our way of dealing with intense feelings. However, this is merely a pattern that doesn't serve us. Instead, it causes us to bottle up emotions so much it can seem too scary to digest them. Once we have learned how to digest strong emotions, however, they can be used as a vehicle to experience life more fully. Pain and pleasure make you feel alive, and that is a beautiful thing. In *yogic* philosophy, one of the layers that connects

Leila Worby

the physical body with the subtle body is the emotional body. We will explore these layers in more detail below. For now, just know you can feed your subtle body and make it more robust through the practice of digesting your emotions. And when you have a strong, subtle body, toxic people won't bother you anymore. You shine, and your inner strength subconsciously attracts other beings. For many people, this is probably the most essential practice for achieving well-being. Usually, it's those strong emotions that stand in the way of attaining actual well-being and equilibrium. I suggest you use the technique outlined above whenever you feel overwhelmed by strong emotions.

According to *Tantric* philosophy there is no right and wrong, no black and white—only shades of grey. Life is just part of the divine play, orchestrated by the divine for it to recognize itself. And everything is part of the divine. With this knowledge, you know that you have nowhere to go, nothing to become. You can just relax into your own true inner essence, your *hridaya*. And let go of trying to become anything because you are already perfect, just as you are. You are divine.

THE PHYSIOLOGY OF THE *PANCHA KOSHAS*

Yogic philosophy outlines the *pancha kosha*, which are five different layers, or sheets of the body, moving from gross to subtle. According to *Classical Hatha Yoga*, the five *koshas* are *annamaya*, *pranamaya, manomaya, vijnanamaya, and anandamaya*. Roughly translated, these are the physical or meat sheet, the life force or vital sheet, the mind sheet, the wisdom sheet, and the bliss sheet.

THE PHYSICAL SHEET—
ANNAMAYA KOSHA

This is the physical meat body, the concrete sheet of the body that all humans are aware of. *Anna* literally means "food" or "physical matter," and "*maya*," in this context, means "to be made of."

It's the body we can feel and touch. The body that can digest food. It consists of the hair, skin, nails, muscles, joints, ligaments, and bones. It's associated with the earth and water elements. The best way to keep this layer happy, healthy, and vibrant is by looking after the needs of the physical body. Healthy living and *yogic* poses are the *yogic* tools to strengthen this sheet.

THE VITAL SHEET— PRANAMAYA KOSHA

Prana means "life force energy." In yoga, we consider the breath a carrier of *prana*. We use *pranayama* to strengthen the *pranamaya kosha*. This layer is considered the physiological, vital, or energetic layer. The flow of our physiological body happens here with the functions of respiration, circulation, and digestion. Because the breath controls the nervous system, the nervous system connects this layer with the *annamaya kosha*, or meat body. This layer is associated with fire and water in *yogic* philosophy.

Because water flows, it makes sense that it would be associated with the circulatory processes of the body. Additionally, in nature, water containing salt acts as a conductor of electricity. Electricity is a concentrated form of life force or *prana*.

Water is furthermore associated with our creative and reproductive power center. To understand the connection between the water element as a *yogic* concept and life force, think of a time when you were physically attracted to another human. There is a reason these encounters are described as "electric" and "magnetic." That energy is the most readily available concentration of life force and can be used as a gateway into the subtle body if it's not physically consummated. But this takes a lot more restraint than *pranayama*, so I recommend starting there when working on strengthening this sheet. To understand how *prana* permeates us from a physiological standpoint you might also consider that oxygen is brought into the body through the breath and is then transitioned into the bloodstream, where it reaches and vitalizes every cell of our being.

Leila Worby

THE MIND SHEET—
MANOMAYA KOSHA

This is the layer of the mind. It's thought of as the psychological layer and the emotional instigator because it contains the endless monologue of the ego. Notice how the mind constantly feeds you the story of your role and perspective in relationships. If you are just a little observant, you are able to separate yourself from these ramblings and realize they are not important to anyone else but you. And as such, they are completely worthless. They are *maya*-an illusion, a cloak of ignorance, to prevent you from experiencing your true divine nature. Which is the realization that you are just a small part of the greater whole of existence. This layer is associated with air and space. To make the most of it and transcend beyond it, you must understand how to master the mind.

The *yogic* tool for mastering the mind is *mantra* recitation. Traditionally you repeat the *mantras* 108 times, using a mala to keep count as you meditate on these sacred sounds. They work to quiet your mind by forcing your mind to focus exclusively on the words or syllables that the *mantra* contains. Focusing your attention on the *mantra* makes the other internal monologue fade out into the background and eventually quiet it altogether. The seed or *bija mantras* outlined later in this book additionally stimulates your energetic body.

The best pose for tuning in and exploring your energetic body is *shavasana* or corpse pose that happens at the end of class. Never skip this one. *Shavasana* is the main pose that allows you to deeply trigger the Parasympathetic Nervous System, and as such, it is the most rejuvenating pose of them all. Don't miss this chance to drop your cortisol levels, increase your metabolism, and increase your serotonin and dopamine (neurotransmitters that increase your happiness and metabolism). *Yoga* can balance your endocrine system if you manage to continuously activate the Parasympathetic Nervous System as a result of a deep, regular practice. The deeper you move into the PNS, the more you relax, and the more the feel-good endorphins will flow.

When people leave *yoga* class before *shavasana* because they think it's merely a resting pose similar to taking a nap, they are missing out on the most potent aspect of *yoga*. They will still reap the blood-moving benefits of *yoga*, but they won't achieve the state of physical finetuning or the surrender necessary to bring the mind and breath to their focused and calm baseline.

THE WISDOM SHEET— VIJNANAMAYA KOSHA

This layer is called the wisdom layer, and it's associated with the element of ether. Once we quiet the mind, the soul can speak. This is where true integrated knowledge and wisdom reside, a place where we start going beyond ourselves and our petty everyday thoughts. If we're lucky, we can tap into the accumulated knowledge of humankind through the pathway of meditation. The *yogic* tool to access this layer is the scriptures or any philosophical or scientific literature. By thirsting for and exploring more universal knowledge than what happens in the realm of the basic mind, we enter the wisdom layer.

THE BLISS SHEET— ANANDAMAYA KOSHA

Ananda means "bliss" in Sanskrit. If you have ever found yourself smiling for no reason at all after *yoga*, you have briefly experienced the bliss layer. An experience of lightness and pure joy of being alive, it is often referred to as the "*yoga* afterglow" by *yoga* practitioners. The *anandamaya kosha* is associated with the ether because it contains all the other elements. Once you have balanced all of the elements, greater influxes of life force will become available to you. And your experience of *ananda* will increase and one day become your normal state of being.

You are able to access the bliss sheet through the other sheets. Once you master *ujjayi* breathing (a *pranayama* described in detail later in this book) as you move through the poses, you may sense blissful and sometimes even ecstatic openings in the subtle body. The breath carries prana and the *ujjayi pranayama* builds up the levels of *prana* and oxygen available to you through the breath. The combination of that pranic build up and the movement of the spine (where the subtle body resides) in all different directions possible during postural practice, stimulates and activates the subtle body. Particularly in the backbends you might experience intense states of euphoria when you pierce through the sheets all the way to the bliss body. These types of experiences usually take years for practitioners to sensitize themselves enough to enjoy. In the beginning it's more a feeling of cleanliness and lightness that continues to pull you back to your *yoga* mat.

Consistent practice of *pranayama* is another tool to discover bliss and ecstasy without having to move your body. The same goes for chanting *mantras*. You are able to stimulate your subtle body all the way into its core, the bliss layer, particularly if you chant with devotion. *Bhatki* (devotional) practices will stimulate the heart center, where the greatest bliss known to mankind resides. Through patiently observing and calming the fluctuations of mind, you are able to reach a place of complete stillness, and from that stillness you can experience the bliss sheet. Everyone who's ever undertaken any scientific endeavor will know the bliss of the eureka state.

Anyone can reach the bliss layer *yogic* practice provides, but the method differs depending on your constitution. Because your constitution determines what kind of method will resonate most profoundly with you. Tapping into the bliss sheet is regarded as tapping into the great all-encompassing soul, the god or goddess of our universe.

THE VAGUS NERVE— THE GATEWAY TO THE SUBTLE BODY

Yogic philosophy teaches us that *prana*, or life force, permeates all five layers of the body. As mentioned before, breath carries *prana*. Breath controls the oxygen levels available to the brain and body as a whole. Oxygen levels greatly impact our vitality and cognition, often allowing us access to the feeling of euphoria.

How we breathe also has a mechanical impact on the nervous system. Breathing causes the diaphragm to physically massage and stimulate the vagus nerve. The longest nerve in the human body, the vagus nerve travels from the brain to the throat and then through the heart and the gut, down to the lumbar spine. It is the main operator of the Parasympathetic Nervous System, and it governs heart activity, digestive functions, and some of the body's main neurological responses, such as mood regulation and brain concentration. The vagus nerve is additionally considered the most essential nerve when it comes to spiritually altered states of consciousness.

In *yogic* philosophy, the spine is regarded as the spiritual body. It may help you to think of the vagus nerve in this way. This explains why, when you experience strong emotion, you often feel a corresponding feeling in the body, such as a pit in your stomach or a tightening of your throat. All strong emotions live along the spine.

Your breath controls and calms the mind by interacting with the vagus nerve. You can calm a stressed state with deep, slow breathing, and with an emphasis on a slow exhalation. This strokes the vagus nerve, which sends a signal to your brain to slow down the nervous system, which in turn slows your agitated state. Conversely, if you are in a state of deep depression, you want to stimulate the vagus nerve by almost giving it *"yogic* CPR" with your diaphragm through more vigorous yet controlled breathing, similar to what is achieved by activating a breathing technique called *bhastrika pranayama**, or breath of fire (a breathing technique that can be dangerous for those with pre-existing heart conditions.) A more subtle breathing practice, safe for all, is *surya bhedana*. *"Surya"* means sun, and *"bhedana"* means to pierce or pass through. It's a warming and activating *pranayama*.

If you have a practice that has allowed you to become centered as you move through life, and your nervous system isn't easily rattled, it can feel good to stimulate the vagus nerve through strong emotion as explained in the previous chapter. It makes you feel alive, and it reaffirms your sense of embodiment. Additionally, stimulation of the vagus nerve will help keep it toned. You can tone it with the breath and by fully feeling your emotions, without holding back. But the moment you give your energy to the story attached to that emotion, you feed the mind layer, or the *manomaya kosha*, which often causes the energy to get stuck, moving you away from your center. You want to move past it by feeding the bliss layer, or *anandamaya kosha*. This can be a blissful full-body experience if you abide in the emotion and completely let go of the story. An excellent practice to distance yourself from the actual stories attached to your feelings is to watch your emotions arise and subside like clouds in the sky. Keep your attention on the clear, blue sky and the movements of the clouds in your peripheral view, knowing they are constantly changing.

Through the simple practice of *pranayama*, it is possible to feel ecstasy or pure bliss. *Yoga* poses create more space for the breath to permeate the body. It usually takes time to access the bliss layer, but for some, it happens directly, almost intuitively.

* Please consult your doctor before adopting variable breathing practices, especially if you suspect you have heart conditions.

THE *GUNAS*—
THE *YOGIC* VIEW ON THE COMPOSITION OF REALITY

Yogic philosophy outlines the different imbalances that cause discord and disease in humans, so you can pinpoint those imbalances and identify the set of techniques that will best support you on your journey toward balance.

In the masterpiece, *Bhagavad Gita*, one of the primary texts of *yogic* philosophy, *Krishna* reveals the nature of reality to *Arjuna*. *Krishna* is the avatar of *Vishnu*, one of the main gods in Hinduism, and in some streams of Hinduism, the central godhead. *Krishna* explains that there are three components to everything, called the *gunas* (qualities or attributes). They are called *sattva*, *rajas*, and *tamas*. From the food we eat to the people we surround ourselves with, the *gunas* are present and make up everything in different measures. You are composed of the *gunas* in unique measurements that change throughout your lifetime, according to how you live your life and what you ingest through your senses. The good news is that there are *yogic* practices that can help you achieve perfect balance for your constitution and situation. To better understand the *gunas*, it is helpful to think of the life stages of a rose. *Sattva* is the perfect pure moment of the blossoming rose. *Rajas* is the force that makes the rose grow from a seed to a budding flower, and *tamas* is the force that causes the flower to wither and die.

SATTVA (PURITY)

Sattva is the divine state of perfect balance and pure consciousness. This is the state *yogis* aspire to cultivate with food, surroundings, and *yogic* practices. When we access this state, we know it. It's when everything is in perfect balance and we are centered and connected with our divine nature. We experience clarity of mind, a wordless pause of truth—the pause between the inhale and the exhale yogis are trained to focus on as a gateway to pure consciousness. The *sattvic* time of day is roughly between 3:30 AM and sunrise. These are magical hours for *yogis*; this is when the ether is calm because people without a spiritual practice are still asleep. Fewer text messages are being sent. It's an easier time of day to cultivate a deeper connection to the all-encompassing life force. Some people like to refer to this concept as god/goddess or all-encompassing soul. In most cultures that teach meditation, the culmination of the practice usually happens just at sunset and sunrise. It is taught that the *sushumna nadi*, the primary energy channel that roughly corresponds to the human body's spine, is open during this time. As such, it's easier to raise energy during these hours. In an ideal world, this is when you want to practice *yoga*.

Sattva is characterized by lightness. I often hear students say they feel so light after class. This is because they are cultivating *sattva* in their bodies. As you continue to practice, you will start craving this lightness. You will intuitively turn toward light foods, such as fresh fruit and vegetables. *Yoga* reinforces lightness throughout all dimensions of your life, from the people you interact with to your food choices.

RAJAS (ACTIVITY)

Rajas is an active, passionate, and competitive force that compels people to achieve. It's the inhalation that marks the beginning. As a positive force, it can be a great force of activation and creativity. However, in its negative, excessive state, it can cause over-activation, leading to rumination, anxiety, panic attacks, and mental instability.

Rajas is active during the morning hours, after sunrise, to midday, the time of day when we are most productive. An overly *rajasic* person is either someone we might consider toxic—prideful, political, and ambitious to an excessive or detrimental degree—or someone suffering from excessive worry, panic, and an inability to structure their thoughts. *Rajas*-inducing foods, such as fish, chicken, anything spicy, wine, and caffeine are activating and stimulating.

TAMAS (DARKNESS AND DESTRUCTION)

The qualities of *tamas* are slow, heavy, dull, and inert. In its full expression, *tamas* is likened to a demonic state of depression and sadness. Its tangible qualities are moist, thick, and compact. You experience *tamas* when you want to roll over in bed and go back to sleep. It's a foggy, tired quality that is hard to shake.

Tamas is most active during the late evening; this is when the body slows down and should rest and prepare to reset. It is during this time we are most likely to indulge in *tamas*-inducing activities, such as drinking alcohol, taking recreational drugs, eating processed foods, and binge-watching Netflix.

Ingestibles that induce *tamas* are red meat, garlic, onions, bread, reheated food, hard alcohol, and marijuana. These foods and substances tend to make us feel sleepy, heavy, and dull. We have all encountered excessively *tamasic* people. They tend to favor the couch over staying active and have a hard time leaving the house or even the bed.

By now, you have probably identified your imbalance and applied the concept of the *gunas* to people in your life, to your lifestyle, and to your food choices. If you are suffering from an abundance of *tamas*, you may need to stimulate *rajas* through *yogic* practices to snap yourself out of your inactive state. And if you are suffering from an excess of *rajas*, you may need to stimulate *tamas* to slow down your mind so you can achieve focus and clarity.

Rajas is pacified through relaxation. Slow down, and reduce things that guide your attention outward as much as you can. Minimize screen time to work hours, and minimize the time you spend in artificial lighting and busy places with many people. Spend time in nature. Spend time in restorative *yoga* poses and in deep meditation. If you don't have a meditative practice, I highly recommend one of the guided meditation apps that are so popular at the moment. Commit to taking a warm bath and going to bed early, listening to a soothing voice as you fall asleep. Avoid spicy food and things that rattle your nervous system, such as caffeine, wine, and strong physical workouts like running, CrossFit, or power *yoga* sessions. If you are a caffeine addict like I am, try to limit your intake to three cups of coffee a day and no stimulants after 5 PM. On the occasions that I drink wine, I only have it with my lunch so it won't interfere with my sleep. Sometimes you will want to socialize and drink in the evenings, but in order to alleviate *rajas*, you should avoid drinking alcohol daily.

Consider your waking hours, and adjust them to rise with the sun and retire with the sunset. Adapt your eating habits to align with *sattvic* foods. Avoid stimulants, or at the very least, cut down on them. Minimize interactions with people who drain you. Assess how you move your body, and if you're *tamasic*, move it more and as vigorously as you can manage. If you're overly *rajasic*, move it less and, more importantly, move it slowly. Turn the senses inward, become meditative, and practice surrender.

How do you fix a *tamasic* imbalance? Because *tamas* is the most serious of the imbalances, I recommend making a substantial change if you can manage it. I am usually a proponent of small shifts that are sustainable, but you don't want to allow yourself to abide in *tamas* for too long as it gets increasingly harder to shift away from this state of deep depression and inactivity. Consider your basic habits and surroundings, and adjust where you can by making more *sattvic* choices. For instance, if you tend to stay up after sunset and drink a lot of alcohol while munching on processed food, try shifting that by cutting out alcohol, fasting after sunset, and going to bed before 10 PM. Set your alarm, and make sure you get out of bed so you can take a few moments to look at the sunrise. Many people keep themselves up late, reasoning they need time to themselves after a full workday. If you crave that time for yourself, start going to bed early and waking up early. Utilize the hours before you have to go to work, and see if that changes anything in your life. This is when your head is clear and you can actually use that time productively. Some of the most successful people in the world make the most of these hours. Examples of heavy hitters that rise before dawn are Michelle Obama (former First Lady of the United States), Jack Dorsey (the CEO of Twitter), and Tim Cook (the CEO of Apple), as well as one of my favorite authors, Ernest Hemingway, who used to create his art at 5 AM.

The above suggestions are strategies that can move you toward a more *sattvic* state. You can also make a plan to get fresh whole foods into your system. Commit to at least an hour-long walk in nature each day, ideally, first thing in the morning, before breakfast if your life allows it.

We will now outline *yogic* techniques and after outlining them all there are curated practices at the end of the book for you to help you pacify a *rajas* or *tamas* imbalance and move towards a more *sattvic* state. As we outline the *yogic* practices we will start with the most powerful technique—the *pranayamas*. If you can only do five minutes of any of the techniques in this book, let it be *pranayama*.

CHAPTER 2

Pranayamas

PRANAYAMA

Pranayama is a Sanskrit word that means "extension of the breath," or more accurately, "extension of life force." *Pranayamas* are *yogic* breathing techniques, used to cultivate life force or *prana*. If I could do only one *yogic* practice a day, I would choose *pranayama*.

The most powerful tool to balance your nervous system is the breath. If you are in a state of profound dissonance, fatigue, or exhaustion, sometimes the only thing you can do is breathe. Breath is available to everyone and can be used to calm or stimulate the nervous system. In my own practice, I prefer to do *pranayama* before *asana* (postural) practice simply because it stabilizes my nervous system immediately and deepens my connection to and enjoyment of the poses. If I don't have time to do *pranayama* before practice, I pay a lot of attention to the *ujjayi pranayama* (explained in detail below) while flowing through poses. Always remember, breath is boss, and the poses are just expressions of the breath.

Yogic scriptures emphasize that one should undertake *pranayama* only with the guidance of a *guru* or enlightened teacher. I recommend finding a teacher who will demonstrate these techniques and observe you in practice. If you can't find one, or can't afford one, go slowly and see how your body feels. Be your own inner *guru*, and stop if you feel uncomfortable. If you are suffering from PTSD, trauma, depression, or any other mental illness, please seek your doctor's and a senior *yoga* teacher's counsel, and only use this book as a supplement to your existing treatment. These practices can help support you on your way back to wellness, but everybody is unique, and what works for some people may be harmful for others. Proceed with caution, and listen to how these practices make you feel.

In traditional *yoga*, we start with the physical practice, the *namaskars* (movement mediations or salutations) and poses, before moving on to *pranayama* (breathing exercises) and meditation. *Namaskars* open the hips and prepare the body to be seated for an extended time.

Since we are trying to establish a balanced nervous system, and we are not coming to this practice to achieve enlightenment, we will start with breathing exercises. We don't need to sit in meditation for hours. We do however need to sit upright, maintaining a straight spine, to open our natural channels of energy to allow life force energy to flow through them freely.

THE FORGOTTEN ART OF SITTING

Before you start any meditation or breathing practice, the most important thing to do is find a way to position your body so your spine is straight. In *Classical Hatha Yoga* many different poses, such as *siddhasana* and *padmasana*, naturally encouraged a straight spine. In fact, almost all the early poses of *Hatha Yoga* were different seated poses. These poses are usually out of reach for contemporary people. We spend too much time sitting in chairs. If you must, and it's the only way to keep your spine straight, sit in a chair to meditate. This should, however, be the last resort.

You may want to consider working on opening your hips to achieve comfort while sitting cross-legged on the earth and maintaining an erect spine. This will prevent lower back pain further down the road. To help straighten the spine in a cross-legged position you want to elevate the sitz bones. You can achieve that by placing a folded blanket under your glutes. If you need to, place rolled up blankets, one between each knee and the ground. You want to feel comfortable and like you could stay seated for as long as you'd like.

Another option for achieving a straight spine while seated is to straddle a big cushion, with your shins and the tops of your feet resting on the earth. I remember feeling frustrated by not being allowed to meditate lying down. *Shavasana* felt so good, and sitting upright took a lot of effort after a while. The reason we sit upright during meditation is to prevent ourselves from falling asleep. We want to maintain a clear and alert state of mind, so we can fully focus our attention.

When we lie down it's easier to descend into a state of total body relaxation, which is a form of rejuvenation that occurs just before we fall asleep. In *tantra* we talk about four states: the awakened state, the deep sleep state, the dreaming state, and *turyia*, or pure consciousness. In some scriptures there is a fifth state called *turiyatita*, which describes the enlightened being that can abide in all states simultaneously. It's said in the scriptures that we pass through *turyia* at the time we awake from sleep. This is also one of the reasons we don't wake meditators up who fall asleep in meditation. We don't want to rob them of the *turyia* experience. Ideally, for meditation, we want to stay awake and alert, so we are able to command the mind and learn how to enter the state of flow with ease and at will.

ESSENTIAL OILS

Essential oils are a way of using nature to support your physical and emotional well-being. You can use them to elevate your mood, move deeper into relaxation, or promote fertility. The possibilities are endless. I particularly enjoy using them just before my *pranayama* practice.

Whenever you create a ritual in your life, anything sensory that is included will remind you of that ritual, allowing you to access the state that the ritual imparts on you. This happens subconsciously, from the smells you smell, to the tastes you taste, to the music you hear. A ritual, refers to every habit or routine you follow, from your daily walk with your dog as you feel the ocean breeze on your cheek, to the smells in the restaurant where you regularly meet your best friend, to the taste of the wine you share with your husband every Friday evening.

I first discovered *yoga's* physical postural practice because my dear friend Caroline took me to a *Bikram Yoga* practice. I fell in love with the practice and stayed with it for years. My constitution runs cold, so I longed for the warmth of the Bikram studio in the evenings. The only thing that dampened my enthusiasm was the smell of sweat and the condensation that happened in the Bikram studio. I simply couldn't stand the smell. I have a big, susceptible nose. I started rubbing lavender scented oil into the palms of my hands, and whenever a feeling of nausea came over me, I inhaled the lavender, and it calmed me. One day while out driving and feeling stressed, I reached for my lavender oil and immediately shifted into the state of flow *yoga* brought me to. My body responded by relaxing, just like the dogs in Pavlov's experiment responded by drooling as their body anticipated food when the bell rang. I like essential oils because they are easy to keep in my purse. Oils have calming properties of their own. You have to establish a practice (for example, twenty minutes of *yoga* and meditation every day or a ninety-minute class three times a week) to access the flow state by smelling a calming scent. Like I mentioned before, you are a product of your habits, and this is a way to make the fruits of your habit—your *yoga* practice—accessible to you instantaneously by simply smelling your essential oils when needed throughout your day.

Leila Worby

Five-Minute *Pranayamas*

UJJAYI BREATHING
(RAJAS PACIFYING)

Ujjayi breathing is also called the "ocean breath," or the "breath of victory." We achieve this breathing by restricting the back of the throat and the vocal cords slightly, creating an ocean-like sound at the back of the throat as the breath flows in and out of the nose. Keeping the mouth genty closed. This extends the breath, allowing us to absorb more oxygen and build up *prana* in our bodies. The goal is to cultivate light *ujjayi* breathing while flowing through *namaskars* and while moving deeper into the poses.

*NADI SHODHANA**
(RAJAS PACIFYING)

Nadi Shodhana is a fundamental *yogic* practice that balances the nervous system. This practice triggers the Parasympathetic Nervous System and cleanses the subtle body's energy channels to prepare it for more life force. It will immediately relax and rejuvenate you, and it is an excellent way to end your day.

Start in a comfortable cross-legged position, keeping the spine straight. Rub your favorite essential oil into your palms, bring them in front of your nose, and take three to five deep breaths. I recommend lavender or sandalwood, or a few drops of both, especially if your practice is toward the end of your day.

Extend the index and middle fingers of your right hand and bring them to your third eye, the space between the eyebrows. Cover the right nostril with the thumb, and inhale slowly and smoothly all the way into your lower belly through the left nostril. Pause briefly and notice the pregnant pause at the top of the breath. Then, cover the left nostril with your ring finger and free your right nostril. Gently exhale through your right nostril and pause briefly at the bottom of the exhale. Inhale through the right nostril and pause at the top of the breath. Cover your right nostril with your thumb and release your left nostril. Gently exhale through your left nostril. Keep your mouth gently closed during this practice. Continue in this way for five to eight rounds. Or set your alarm for five minutes. I like to use the app *Insight Timer*, because it features soft gong sounds when you have completed your practice. It's less jarring to the nervous system than traditional alarm sounds.

You want to cultivate a feeling of drinking your breath. Every time you breathe, you are filling yourself up with life force. As you cover your nostrils with your fingers, try placing the fingers as high as you can on the nose ridge so you don't make the nostrils stick together. If you would like to deepen this practice, especially if you are a visual practitioner, you can visualize drinking the cool, calming lunar energies and light through your left nostril and the vital, warm, radiating solar energies through your right nostril. This will enhance your experience within the *pranayama*.

* Should you have a stuffy nose, I recommend blowing it and investing in a neti pot to clean it out even further, should you need to. A neti pot is similar to a teapot that can be filled with lukewarm, lightly salted water, for the purpose of rinsing the nasal passages. Pour the fluid into each nostril and let it drain out through the other. This practice clears out mucus and makes it easier to breathe fully.

VILOMA PRANAYAMA
(RAJAS PACIFYING)

Start in a comfortable cross-legged position, keeping the spine straight. Start by rubbing your favorite essential oil into your palms. Bring them in front of your nose, and take three to five deep breaths. For a *rajas* imbalance, I recommend rose, lavender, and sandalwood.

To immediately drop deeply into yourself, I recommend the *viloma* breathing technique. *Viloma* means "against the hair," or to interrupt the breath on the inhale. Start by taking a full deep normal breath.

Exhale fully. As you inhale, drink the breath and stop at the throat. Pause here for a quiet count of three. Then, fill up even more to the heart center, feeling the ribcage expand. Pause here for a count of three. Now fill up all the way into the lower belly as deeply as possible without straining. Pause the breath here for a count of three. Then, softly, smoothly exhale all the air out, using light *ujjayi* breathing. This is one round. Continue like this for five minutes.

Once breathing practices become part of your daily routine, you should be able to tap into them easily. Over time, they will make you more relaxed and able to cope with stress and anxiety. Suppose you are suffering from a panic attack. You may wish to start breathing deeply, focusing on being present and noticing the details of your surroundings. If that doesn't work to ease your anxiety, you can try manipulating the breath to trigger the Parasympathetic Nervous System through *viloma* or *nadi shodhana pranayama*. Please listen profoundly to your response, and only proceed with these techniques if they calm you down. Do not force them if they create more stress.

SQUARE BREATHING
(RAJAS PACIFYING)

This breathing technique is wonderful for dispelling *rajas*. It grounds you deeply into your body, calming and quieting the mind so your soul can speak. I like to use this technique to overcome binge eating or other obsessive, addictive behaviors, because it trains your brain to put one foot in front of the other, which can feel nearly impossible when you are overcome with desire for your favorite food or poison. Incorporate square breathing into your everyday practice, ideally first thing in the morning. Once you have trained your brain to fully integrate this *pranayama*, you will be able to end a relapse before it even begins.

Sit up straight, either cross-legged or straddling a pillow. Rub some of your favorite calming essential oil between the palms. To move toward a healthy eating pattern, I recommend rose and sandalwood or lavender and sandalwood. Take a few deep breaths, savoring the scent of the oil. Begin your *pranayama* by slowly exhaling all of your air out. Gently inhale through your nose to a slow count of four. Pause at the top of the inhale for a count of four. Gently exhale through your nose for a count of four. At the bottom of the exhale, pause and hold for a count of four. Continue for five minutes. As you get more and more used to this technique, you can increase to counts of ten. Go only as far as feels comfortable. This is meant to feel pleasant and relaxing. If you wish, you may add *ujjayi* breathing when doing this *pranayama*.

BHRAMARI PRANAYAMA*, OR "BUMBLEBEE BREATH" (RAJAS AND INSOMNIA PACIFYING)

Rajas can manifest as racing thoughts that make it close to impossible to turn off your mind and go to sleep, let alone structure your day. It is easy to lie awake in the wee hours thinking about the following day's interactions, the emails you need to send first thing in the morning, or the bills you have to pay. To settle your mind, try the *bhramari pranayama*, also known as the "bumblebee breath."

Start in a comfortable cross-legged position, keeping the spine straight. Spread your shoulders wide. Now open your palms and close your ears with your thumbs. Place your index fingers on your forehead, right above your eyebrows. Let the middle finger and ring finger gently rest on top of your closed eyes. Breathe deeply and slowly, and on the exhale, make a humming sound. Your fingers should feel the vibration as they rest on your face. Continue this way for seven repetitions. Then, gently remove your hands from your face and rest them on your lap.

You may work your way up to seventeen repetitions, adding one repetition each round as you feel ready. Once you have completed this *pranayama*, take a few moments to really feel how your physical, emotional, and subtle body responds to this practice.

* *Bhramari* should not be practiced by pregnant or menstruating women. It is also contraindicated for high blood pressure, epilepsy, chest pain, or an active ear infection. *Bhramari* should be practiced in a seated position.

BHASTRIKA PRANAYAMA,*
OR "BREATH OF FIRE" (TAMAS PACIFYING)

Bhastrika pranayama, also known as "breath of fire," is considered the most powerful *pranayama* of *yoga*. It works to strengthen, awaken, and supercharge your nervous system by clearing obstacles and breathing life into your being. Ideally, you would do five minutes of *nadi shodhana*, followed by five minutes of *bhastrika*. However, if you only have five minutes, start with this. Your breath will work as energetic CPR, bringing you back to life again, and soon, you will have more energy to undertake more practices.

Start in a comfortable cross-legged position, keeping the spine straight. Rub your favorite essential oil into your palms, bring them in front of your nose, and take three to five deep breaths. For a *tamas* imbalance, I recommend tangerine or lemongrass. Any citrus smell, such as grapefruit or lemon, is good. Orange is good for depression. Pick one and use it to create a conditioning effect, in which the scent triggers your natural response, and let the inherent properties of the essential oils aid your mood.

Now, observe the breath for a few rounds until it flows deeply and smoothly on its own. Take a deep breath through the mouth. Then, breathing through the nose, start pumping the diaphragm in and out, making a sniffing sound. Similar to the sound a dog makes when it is trying to discern a specific smell. The inhale and exhale must be equally as long. Make your breaths deep enough to make your belly button dance and your stomach pulse out on the inhale, and in on the exhale. After five minutes of breathing like this, draw as much air as you can into the lungs, and then sip in even more air. Hold the breath here as long as it feels manageable, squeezing your perineum and anus as hard as you can. This is called *moola bandha*, or the root lock, in *yoga*, and it keeps the energy in you and ultimately shifts the energy upward through you to energize your entire being. Once you have mastered the root lock, you may add *uddiyana bandha*, or the abdominal lock, by pulling the navel to the spine simultaneously as you engage the root lock. This requires quite a lot of control, but I encourage you to explore it once you feel comfortable with the root lock.

* If you are suffering from any heart problems or elevated blood pressure, or if you are pregnant or menstruating, please do not undertake this *pranayama*. Instead, do *surya bhedana pranayama*, as outlined below.

SURYA BHEDANA PRANAYAMA
(TAMAS PACIFYING)

A more subtle way of awakening the inner sun is by activating the right *nadi* through *surya bhedana pranayama*. The right *nadi* is called *pingala*. A masculine, radiating, strong, and physical power channel, it is associated with the sun.

To assist with this *pranayama*, place the index finger and middle finger of the right hand between the eyebrows, then use the ring finger to close off the left nostril for inhalation through the right nostril. Hold the breath for as long as is comfortable. Then, close off the right nostril with the thumb, and lift the ring finger to allow full exhalation through the left nostril. Close the left nostril with the ring finger as you remove the thumb from the nose and inhale through the right nostril. Notice the pause at the top of the breath. Continue in this way for five minutes, keeping the mouth gently closed.

CHAPTER 3

Mantras, Mudras, and Meditation

MANTRAS

The word "*mantra*" is derived from two Sanskrit words—*manas* (mind) and *tra* (tool). "*Mantra*" literally means "a tool for the mind." *Mantras* are designed to replace the chatter of the mind and achieve focused attention that will allow the practitioner to transition into deep meditation. They bring the mind under control. They are traditionally repeated 108 times.

The *bija mantras* that will be outlined later in this book, are seed *mantras* that stimulate the *chakras*. They will awaken your energetic body and circulate the life force in you. It's one of the most powerful practices to undertake, and it's not advisable to do so until you have balanced your nervous system.

As a side note, beyond the scope of this book, there are *mantras* in the *tantric* traditions that are considered deities in sound form. And they form the foundation for *tantric* deity meditations. The *tantric* tradition is sometimes referred to as "the path of the *mantras.*" Please don't confuse *mantras* with New Age affirmations such as "I am happy this morning" that you write on a Post-it and stick to your mirror to improve your mood. In *yoga*, *mantras* are considered sacred vibrations that profoundly impact your energy body and can work both for protection and transformation.

THE *GAYATRI MANTRA* FOR FOCUSED AND INCREASED ENERGY (*SATTVA* PROMOTING)

The most powerful of all *mantras*-the *Gayatri*, is the root (most foundational) *mantra* of *yogic* practices. It's outlined in the *Rig Veda*, the oldest of the *Vedas*. The *Vedas* are religious scriptures dated between 1500–1200 BCE. We honor the sun and bring light into every facet of our lives by chanting the *Gayatri Mantra* every morning at sunrise eleven times. This practice will reconstruct the daily dialogue that happens in your mind. It will eliminate toxic chatter and enhance positive beliefs. The real *yoga* is to learn not to believe your thoughts and to slow them down. The *Gayatri* will help with both. This *mantra* impacts emotional well-being and offers strong protection, should you need it. It will help you turn your attention and perception toward the light.

Whenever you feel like you are in a state of despair, turn this *mantra* on. Choose your favorite recording, there are many beautiful versions of this *mantra* on spotify, and chant along with them. That's a good way to learn the pronunciation of Sanskrit words initially. Allow it to bring you back to the peacefulness and clarity of mind you experienced when you chanted it at sunrise. If you suffer from excessive worrying and anxiety, please turn to the *Gayatri*. Let it help you free your mind of words, turning the chatter into the gentle chanting of *Gayatri* as it moves you from darkness to light.

The *mantra*

AUM, Bhur Bhuva Suvah. Tat Savitur Varenyam. Bhargo Devasya Dhimahi. Dhiyo Yo Nah. Prachodayat.

The meaning of the *Gayatri Mantra*

We meditate on that most adored Supreme Lord, the creator, whose effulgence (divine light) illuminates all realms (physical, mental, and spiritual). May this divine light illuminate our intellect.

SOHAM KRIYA FOR FOCUSED ATTENTION (RAJAS PACIFYING)

There are two ways of doing this *kriya*. The first one will bring you into the moment, allowing you to drop into your body in deep communion with your breath.

SOHAM FOR BODY AWARENESS

Simply come to your comfortable cross-legged position with an erect spine. As you inhale, gently whisper the sound *SO* on the inhale and *HAM* on the exhale. Pause at the top of the inhale, and also at the bottom of the exhale, making these pauses as long as it feels natural and right. Work on breathing deeply and slowly. You may wish to add *ujjayi pranayama* to this *kriya*.

SOHAM FOR FOCUSED ATTENTION

The second way to do this *kriya* awakens your third eye *chakra* and creates a razor-like focus. Visualize a *bindu* (small focal point) made out of pure light, almost like a small full moon, and pull it in through your third eye, the point between your eyebrows, all the way down to the base of your spine, as you chant *SO* internally. Pause the breath here for as long as feels good, gently squeezing your pelvic floor and anal muscles, known as the root lock, or *moolah bandha*, in *yoga*. Exhale as you let go of the contraction, visually moving the *bindu* all the way up your spine and out through the third eye, internally chanting *HAM*. I enjoy doing this *kriya* under the full moon and using it as an external focal point that moves up and down my spine. The spine again, in *yogic* philosophy, is where the subtle body lives. And this *kriya* will activate it.

OMKAR KRIYA
(TAMAS PACIFYING)

This is one of the most powerful *kriyas* of *yoga*. It allows you to connect and vibrate with life force. By practicing this *kriya* three times in a row, you will feel activated, peaceful, and meditative.

Start in a cross-legged position, keeping the spine erect. Take three mindful breaths. Take a breath and exhale it fully. Then, inhale deeply, and on the exhale, make the sound *AAAAAAAAHH*, focusing on your solar plexus center, which is the area just below your sternum, also known as the *manipura chakra*. Take five breaths each time, exhaling *AAAAAHH*. On your sixth inhale, focus your attention on your heart center, and make the sound *UUUUUUHH*. Do this for five breaths. Then move your attention to your throat and exhale the sound *MMMMMMHH* for five rounds. Lastly, shift your attention to the crown, or more specifically the space just one or two inches above your crown, as you make the sound *AUM* five times, letting the vibrations emanate from your crown center. See if you can bring the tip of your tongue to the roof of your mouth and close the ears while resounding the *AUM* internally. Repeat this *kriya* three times. It will make you vibrate with life force.

ASATOMA SADGAMAYA MANTRA
FOR THE SOLAR JUNCTIONS

This *mantra* is a humble prayer and a reminder to turn toward the light, to not lose track of your spiritual practice in favor of your worldly duties and desires. I recommend it for solar junction practices because it helps with starting a new cycle. It's furthermore an invocation of light, which is needed during the winter solstice, and it is a wonderful way to honor and embrace the abundance of light that we get to enjoy during the summer solstice.

The *mantra*

AUM Asato Ma Sadgamaya, Tamaso Ma Jyotir Gamaya, Mrityormaamritam Gamaya. AUM. Shanti, Shanti, Shanti.

The meaning of the *Asatoma Sadgamaya Mantra*

From ignorance, lead me to truth. From darkness, lead me to light, and from death lead me to immortality. AUM. Peace, peace, peace.

There are some really lovely *mantras* to listen to and flow to during the time of the new moon. One of my personal favorites is the *Adi Shakti mantra*, an invocation to the primordial mother and the creative life force, from the *Kundalini Yoga* tradition. It's nice to listen to during the dark moon because she is hiding, so this moon phase evokes a longing for her and a wish to call on her to reenter your life.

This *mantra* is further thought to eliminate fear and fulfill the longings and the desires of the heart. It is said to give you the power to act by removing insecurities that block action.

Listening to the *Adi Shakti mantra* may help heal feelings of loss and abandonment regarding our biological mothers. It helps women connect with the universal and archetypal mother. In many traditions the life force energy is considered a feminine deity that is to be honored, and invoked if you're lucky. It is experienced by humbly chanting her names in reverence. This whole *mantra* consists of her different names and Namo means "to bow to" in Gurmukhi, the language used in this tradition. It's like you're respectfully calling on her for her to enter and bless your life.

The *mantra*

> *Adi Shakti, Namo Namo,*
> *Sereb Shakti, Namo Namo,*
> *Pritam Bhagvati, Namo Namo,*
> *Kundalini, Mata Shakti, Namo Namo!*

The meaning of the *Adi Shakti Mantra*

> *I bow to the primal power*
> *I bow to the all-encompassing power*
> *I bow to the creative power at the beginning*
> *I bow to the divine mother of all peace*

PURNAMADAH MANTRA FOR THE FULL MOON

One of my favorite *mantras* for the full moon is *Purnamadah*. This peace *mantra* awakens and connects you to the radiant fullness that is you and the creative force at play all around you. That is clearly visible during the time of the full moon. It allows for you to bask in your own divine glory through the glory of the full moon.

The *mantra*

Aum.

Purnamadah Purnamidam.

Purnaat Purna-mudacyate.

Purnasya Purna-maadaaya Purnamevaa-vashisyate.

Aum. Shanti, Shanti, Shanti.

The meaning of the *Purnamadah* Mantra

All is full and abundant, always.

This, all that is within you, and that, all that is around you, is fullness.

From that fullness, fullness is forever born again.

Remove fullness from fullness and still, only fullness remains.

Peace, peace, peace!

MUDRAS

Mudras are hand gestures. They are used in *yoga* to move deeper into meditation. They are also used to raise life force. The *mudras* are seals of energy, and they are just as crucial as poses. Poses, essentially, are full-body *mudras*. We have many nerve endings and energy channels in our hands and fingers, so the hands play a vital part in sealing the life force energy and keeping it within. We stimulate different areas of the brain by bringing the tips of different fingers together. I recommend a five-minute *mudra* practice. Usually, *mudras* are held for a minimum of five minutes, lasting up to an hour. Outside of my practice, I like to hold them whenever I'm stuck in a boring place. Sometimes I hold *mudras* in my pockets. My favorite place to practice *mudras* is on the beach. Another set of *mudras* is used in classical Indian temple dance. They express emotions, events, or even creatures. Here, we will focus on the transformative *mudras* of *yoga*.

Five-Minute *Mudra* Practices

SVABHAVA MUDRA FOR CONNECTING WITH YOUR INNER ESSENCE (*SATTVA* PROMOTING)

There are several beautiful *mudras* that we practice in *yoga* to stimulate the subtle body in different ways. One of my absolute favorites is the *svabhava mudra*, which allows you to connect with your true inner essence, the divine essence that encompasses everything. That essence is beyond the chatter of the mind and beyond your physical body. We come to *yoga* to establish this connection.

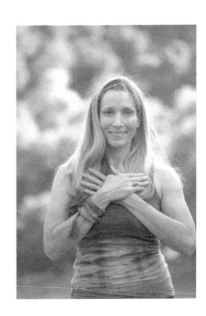

With your palms facing your heart center, simply cross your thumbs, with the right wrist on top of the left. Then, draw the palms of your hands to your chest and rest them there. If you wish to, you can draw a couple of circles over your heart center with the cupped palms of your hands before settling into this practice. Let the breath ebb and flow, naturally deepening on its own.

APAN VAYU MUDRA FOR ELIMINATING PANIC ATTACKS
(RAJAS PACIFYING)

Apan vayu mudra calms the body, regulates the heart, and wards off panic attacks. This *mudra* helps provide space for greater internal awareness and stillness. It invites body-based relaxation and cardiovascular strengthening.

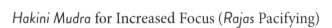

Bend the index finger so the tip curls in and touches the inner web of the thumb. Bring the tips of the middle and ring fingers so they touch the tip of the thumb. Extend the little finger out. Sitting cross-legged, position both hands in this *mudra*, and rest the backs of the hands on your knees while you focus on taking full, deep breaths. If half lotus pose, or even full lotus pose, is comfortable and good for you, take it. If not, just sit in a comfortable cross-legged position, keeping your spine straight.

Hakini Mudra for Increased Focus (*Rajas* Pacifying)

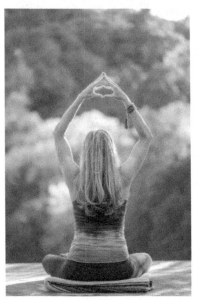

Hakini mudra, also called the "*mudra* for the mind," activates the third eye center to calm and quiet the mind. Useful for improving memory and focus, *hakini mudra* helps you absorb information and maintain concentration for extended periods.

Bring the palms together, a few inches apart. Bring the fingertips and thumbs of both hands together, allowing them to maintain light contact. Then, raise the thumbs to the level of the third eye *chakra*, the center of the forehead. To enhance this *mudra's* benefits, lift the *drishti* (gaze) toward the third eye while breathing through the nostrils. I like to hold the hands at the level with the third eye as long as possible and then rest the wrists and forearms on my thighs, while maintaining my hands in the shape of the *mudra* until my practice is complete.

Leila Worby

PRANA MUDRA*
(TAMAS PACIFYING)

Prana means "life force." This *mudra* is used to awaken, increase, and circulate the life force within you. This is a beautiful *mudra* for dispelling *tamas*.

Come to a comfortable seated position with your spine straight. Bring the attention to your breath as it settles. Gently place the ring finger and little finger at the thumb's tip, and keep the other two fingers stretched out. Rest the backs of your hands on your thighs. Breathe, and let the life force permeate you.

SURYA MUDRA*
(TAMAS PACIFYING)

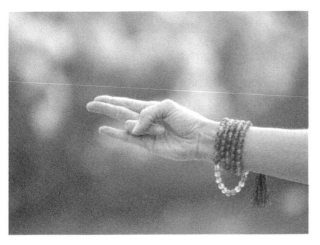

Surya means "sun." This *mudra* is used to ignite the inner sun, the digestive fire. If you have problems with your metabolism and digestion and are feeling sluggish, this is the best *mudra* for you. It will stoke your inner heat.

Bend the ring fingers, and place their tips at the bases of the thumbs. Gently press the thumbs on top of the ring fingers. This pacifies the earth element residing in the ring fingers while increasing the fire element residing in the thumbs.

* For the *prana* and *surya mudras* above, choose the one you feel is best for your circumstances. Do you feel fatigued or sluggish? Do you need to increase life force or do you need to increase the digestive fire (referring here to both emotional digestion and physical body digestion). Practice your chosen *mudra* for at least thirty days before trying the other.

SHAKTI MUDRA FOR FERTILITY

One of my favorite *mudras* for balancing the reproductive system and solving trauma or shame concerning sexuality is *shakti mudra*. It's also a powerful *mudra* that balances the brain hemispheres and brings your masculine and feminine energies into harmony. It can help with PMS or hormonal imbalances in the female system.

Come to a comfortable cross-legged position, keeping your spine straight. Simply wrap the index and middle finger over your thumb. Bring the knuckles and the fronts of the index and middle finger together as you extend the little finger and the ring finger letting the tips of the extended fingers touch. Bring the *mudra* to your lower belly and hold it for five minutes to an hour, allowing the breath to rise and subside as it wants to.

YONI MUDRA FOR FERTILITY

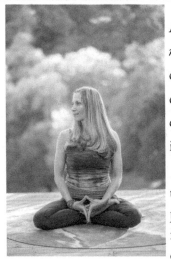

Another *mudra* for supporting fertility and the female body is *yoni mudra*. It allows you to move inward and connect with the origins of creation, the divine feminine, and the womb of humanity. It relaxes and connects you with the deep mysteries of creation and birth. It is also an excellent *mudra* for supporting the already pregnant body and preparing it to give birth.

Start in a comfortable seated position. Bring the tips of your thumbs and the tips of your index fingers together, letting the thumbs point up, and the index fingers point toward the earth, so that they form a womb-like gesture. Interlace the rest of the fingers and rest the outside edges of your hands on the lower belly.

I love this *mudra* because it cultivates unshakable inner trust and confidence. When we struggle to overcome addiction and self-destructive behaviors, we sometimes need to overcome the painful distrust and lack of confidence that stem from lack of connectedness with our true inner essence. We must move deeper to fully inhabit our bodies, which are just temporary dwellings after all. The appearance of your physical body does not determine your value, but it is natural and healthy to maintain your body, making it a clean, cozy dwelling for your soul.

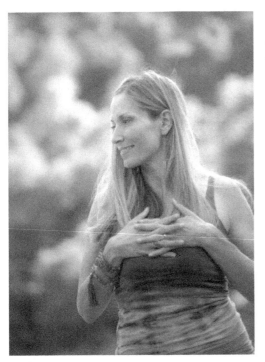

To perform this *mudra*, sit with an erect spine. Rub your hands together until you have created a sensation of heat between your palms. Then interlace your fingers, leaving the thumbs free. Place your palms over your heart center, and simply be with your breath.

It is not uncommon for strong, seemingly unmanageable emotions to boil up when you practice this *mudra*. Should you experience overwhelming emotion, disconnect your story from the feeling. Get to know the emotion. What color is the emotion? What is its shape? How does it impact you physically? Draw the emotion into the core of your being, and absorb it until it disintegrates and passes through you as energy that feeds your energy body, making you healthy and strong.

If you continue to experience overwhelming emotions in this *mudra*, practice the *bhumisparsa mudra* (explained in detail below) until you feel you have processed all, or most, of the overwhelming emotions.

BHUMISPARSA MUDRA* TO AID DIGESTION OF STRONG EMOTIONS

Place your left hand over your heart center and your right hand on the earth. As you inhale, visualize all the sorrow, sadness, and pain flowing from the cave behind your heart into your left hand. Pause the breath here for as long as it feels comfortable while you are collecting energy. Perhaps it has the color of smoke, or maybe it's black or red. Visualize pushing the energy out through your right arm, and eventually through the palm of your right hand, deep into the earth, on the exhale. Stay in this *mudra* while paying attention to your heart center for five minutes.

* Please note that this is a variation of the original *bhumisparsa mudra*. It is more aimed at soothing the emotional body, unlike the original, which is used for spiritual awakening.

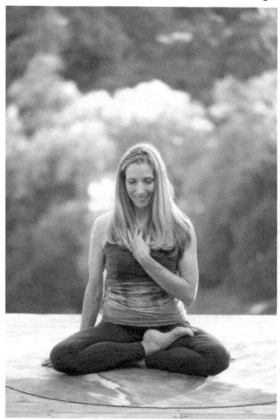

Leila Worby

MEDITATION

Meditation is any activity that allows you to shift your brain waves into *alpha*, or if you're lucky, *theta* brain waves. We meditate for many different reasons: to trigger the PNS and lower stress levels; to overcome trauma; to achieve a more powerful instant recharge; to sharpen our edge and enhance our performance; to achieve deeper orgasms; or to help induce lucid dreaming. The reasons for and possibilities of meditation are endless.

In *yoga*, meditation is used as a vehicle to progressively move from a state of crude human consciousness to one of an enlightened being. There are different kinds of meditation. The more accessible meditation techniques for beginners are awareness cultivation, focus cultivation, and full-body relaxation. In the beginning, the easiest way to achieve a meditative state is to cultivate awareness while moving the body. You can do this when walking or practicing poses by simply slowing down your pace of movement and taking in as much as you can through your senses.

In *yoga*, focus works as a segway into the meditative state. The poses of *yoga* are designed to withdraw your senses and find an inner *drishti* (*drishti* means gaze, but in this context more like a focal point). Every pose or transition in *yoga* has a point in the body where you rest your attention, and through that focus, your consciousness flows into a state of meditation. In the beginning, this focal point is the place where you feel the stretch or contraction in your physical body. This is partly what makes *asana* practice or any type of movement meditation superior to other forms of exercise. It's designed to move you deeply into meditation while you exercise.

Some of the *SOHAM kriya* outlined earlier contains visualization, another type of meditation. Visualization can be used quite successfully after full-body relaxation to soothe the emotional body. Typically by visualizing a soothing environment and a soothing activity in said environment. Spiritual meditations in *yoga*, sometimes known as *kriyas* (actions) are typically a combination of some or all of the following complementary meditation techniques: visualization, *mantra*, *mudra*, *asana* and *pranayama*. Their goal is enlightenment.

WALKING MEDITATION
(*RAJAS* AND *TAMAS* PACIFYING)

Walk mindfully and slowly, so you can allow the movement to become meditative. Focus on the soles of your feet as they touch the earth. Notice the breeze on your cheek and the light coming through the trees. Notice the smells. Become absorbed in your environment. Try to slow down so much that you are able to space out your thoughts and abide in the space between the words and the space between the trains of thought. You want to move your body and your thoughts into a mode of slow motion.

MEDITATING ON THE ELEMENTS
(*RAJAS* AND *TAMAS* PACIFYING)

During your walking meditation and as you move through your day, select one of the elements to notice and on which to focus your senses. If you choose earth, for example, focus on how it feels under your feet, and discern its smell. You can touch it and practice seeing and sensing it wherever it appears. Look at or feel the texture of earth in a flower pot or of the rock formations in your garden, or of the sand at the beach. Notice the smell of earth. Also, work on noticing the incredible power of gravity and how it impacts your being. The same can be done with the other elements as well. The element you choose to focus your attention on determines which *guna* you're pacifying. Consider again that focused attention is a segway into meditation and focusing your attention on your chosen element will additionally help stimulate your subtle body as the element exists within you. You will find more detailed instruction on how to meditate on the respective elements in the chapter "The Elements—Living in flow with nature."

Leila Worby

FULL-BODY AWARENESS AND RELAXATION
(*RAJAS PACIFYING*)

Find a comfortable seated pose that allows for a straight spine. Then, spend five minutes letting your breath flow without controlling it whatsoever. Notice everything about your body. Start from the toes. Notice what it's like to have feet. Notice your ankles, the calves, the shins. Notice your knees, the backs of your thighs, and your quads. Bring your attention to your pelvic bowl, your glutes, and your lower belly. Notice everything about your sacrum and lower back, as well as the front of your torso. Notice your chest, your upper back, and shoulders. Notice your throat, neck, and skull. Notice your entire face, your chin, your cheeks, nose, and forehead.

After you have scanned your whole body from toes to head, bring your attention back to your breath. Let it become automatic, and simply observe it. Rest safely in the knowledge that everything is just perfect and exactly as it should be.

FIRE GAZING
(*RAJAS PACIFYING*)

Since the beginning of time, mankind has relaxed and reposed in front of the home fire. Gazing into a fireplace immediately slows your heart rate and thoughts. It can be used as a gateway into deeper trance states if they are of interest. Please remember, though, that *yoga* happens in all states, not just trance states.

TRATAKA ON CANDLE
(*RAJAS PACIFYING*)

This is one of my favorite practices because it's both calming and centering. Light a candle, and place it on a chair in front of you. Position the flame at the same height as your third eye, the point between your eyebrows. Gaze at the candle, placing all of your attention on the flame. Let yourself be absorbed by it for as long as possible without blinking. Try to focus your attention on the flame to such an extent that you can visually drag it inside you, into your core, where you become one with the light of the candle. Practice gazing at the candle while breathing smoothly and deeply for five minutes. This will allow a massive reset of your nervous system and your ability to focus and stay concentrated for more extended amounts of time.

LIGHT MEDITATION (*TAMAS PACIFYING*)

You may also consider meditating on light. This is particularly useful if you're suffering from depression. This ancient meditation technique shifts your focus, your state of mind, and the state of your entire being toward the light. Notice the light when it shines through the spaces between tree leaves and when it reflects off of ocean waves. See how the sun continues to light up your surroundings as it rises in the morning. Train your mind to always acknowledge and turn toward the light. Once our attention is absorbed by light, darkness is dispelled.

MEDITATION ON THE VOID (BEYOND BALANCING THE GUNAS)

This meditation should ideally follow full-body relaxation. Many of us have accessed this state in *Shavasana*, or upon waking or just as we're going to sleep. During the void state, our hearing is the dominant sense. It's a keen listening to and merging with the silence that encompasses and contains all the noises that surround you. When we attune ourselves to the void, we can sense an all-encompassing presence. When we relax even more and move deeper into this state we can sometimes feel like we have ceased to exist and as if we have been swallowed up by this restful, soothing ocean of darkness. This state is very similar to deep, dreamless sleep, yet we are fully conscious.

Leila Worby

GODDESS MEDITATION
(BEYOND BALANCING THE *GUNAS*)

Goddess meditation is meditation on the divine feminine and can be a life-transforming practice. A critical component of *yoga* is to bring your consciousness into a state that simulates being in the womb to achieve involution, a journey of the soul all the way back to where it began, inside the mother. The womb state we experience as embryos is the first experience we have of the void. This may be why we sometimes associate our *yoga* teachers with mother or father figures. When *yoga* is actually working, we are in a vulnerable state of journeying back into the void, into that experience of our true inner essence.

Because people are not perfect, most of us didn't have perfect parents to support us on our journey through life. The *yoga* journey can be a journey toward revisiting this vulnerable state, with the support of the great mother, through this meditation. When I say "the great mother" I am referring to the archetypal mother figure that is prevalent in all cultures from the dawn of mankind. Experiencing unconditional acceptance and love can be incredibly healing for people who never received those qualities from their birth mother and for those who grew up without a mother. *Yoga* also provides a connection with the divine that supports us in waking up to fully experience the nature of our divine inner essence.

It's nice to do this meditation when you have settled deeply into flow at the end of your practice. Sit with a straight spine in any position that feels good to you. Imagine a motherly, warm, kind, and loving female presence behind you, energetically hugging you from behind. This warm female presence is a divine light figure, and she accepts and loves you exactly as you are. It's an exchange of complete acceptance and soothing. You can feel her heart center connecting with yours through a beam of light. Your heart center is located in a cave just behind your heart, and the goddess mother is filling it with the divine light of love, acceptance, and bliss. She protects you and fills you with love, joy, and delight. If you're on the *yogic* path, you may visualize her as one of the versions of *Shakti*, the divine feminine, that appeals to you in this tradition. If you are more connected to Christianity, you can visualize her as Mother Mary or an angel of protection.

If you're from an Islamic background, Fathma might come alive for you. There is nothing right or wrong. Choose what feels most suitable and natural to you based on your conditioning. She was always there, you see, from the beginning of mankind, throughout all religions and cultures. In the same way there are different words for "love" in the different languages of the world, the divine feminine goes by many different names.

TANTRIC MEDITATION ON NON-DUALITY (BEYOND BALANCING THE GUNAS)

This mediation is best done under the guidance of an experienced *yoga* teacher who has studied and practiced *tantra* for years. You should only attempt it if you are at a very mentally stable place in your life. It's an advanced practice and should only be attempted after you have achieved complete balance through the practices described to balance the *gunas* in this book.

Most people think about sex when they think about *tantra*, but the other side of the *tantra* coin is death. Think of sexual energy as a vibrating aliveness, or as the creative uprising and dynamic energy available to humans. This life force energy springs forth from absolute stillness. One can't have a full-body orgasm without first being able to fully relax past the point of surrender. Death is complete relaxation and deep rest. It's letting go into a stillness, tangible in the meditative state previously defined as *the void*. To access this state, you need to completely surrender to transform. This practice is, to mystics, one of the most extraordinary journeys and methods of meditation.

I like to practice this meditation to the beat of Shamanic drumming on the full moon and during the summer solstice after I have saged myself and the space. Do your practice: *pranayama*, asana, *mantra*, *mudra*, and meditation. Then, come into a very comfortable supine position. You will stay here for thirty to forty minutes. I love Shamanic drumming for journeying while doing this. It helps bring you into deeper states of relaxation. Visualize how your body dies, rotten and decayed until only the bones are left. The bones disintegrate. The remains are blown away by the wind and returned gently to the earth.

For a long while, you will feel that your consciousness is much bigger than just your body. You are part of the nature that surrounds you. Your breath is the wind in the trees. Your body is now the earth. You are part of a vast consciousness, the stillness that contains all sound. Rest in this stillness for a long time, and then slowly start visualizing a new *lightbody*, a body that is perfect, shiny, divine, and created from the pearly white light of the moon. Eventually, your new Lightbody gets bones, flesh, and skin, and a new *you* appears from the elements. This mediation helps you experience the void, the great divine consciousness that is part of everything. It enables you to discover your true nature as one already perfect in its connectedness to the greatness of the whole, the all-encompassing consciousness, known to some of us as god/goddess consciousness. This *tantric* meditation on non-duality is one of the most profound meditations available. It should only be attempted after years of practice. Non-duality is the experience of intimacy with all things. A sense of being part of the whole universe. The sense of being the observer vanishes completely and instead you feel yourself to be whatsoever you are observing. You don't see the ocean, you are the ocean. You don't hear the ocean waves, you are the sound of them crashing against the shore.

CHAPTER 4

The Elements

LIVING IN FLOW WITH NATURE

Cultivating a regular *yoga* practice is one way to live in flow with nature. Living in flow with nature also means enjoying the fresh air, the sun and rain, and the invigorating smells and sounds of the world outdoors. Creating practices that harness and support nature's energies allows you to further drop into the cycles of nature and benefit from their healing effects on your body.

To the ancient *yogi*s, one of the primary practices was to meditate on the elements of nature. These practices are outlined in the *Shiva* and *Gheranda Samhita*, amongst other scriptures. In *yogic* philosophy, the body is considered to be the micro-cosmos that mirrors the macro-cosmos. The spine is the core of the subtle body, with many energetic vortices, referred to as *chakras* that run through it. Each of these energy hubs represents one of the five elements: earth, water, fire, wind, and ether. They run from the base of the spine, which is the seat of our earth center, up through the crown of the head, where we connect with the ether. The elements of nature are essential in *yogic* practices. It's taught in *yogic* philosophy that, through communion with the elements, we can fully experience the divine. This occurs through involution, a movement from the most physical external expression—in this case, the elements, or *pancha bhutas*—to the most ethereal, subtle realm of white light.

When you go on that once a year beach or ski vacation, you may notice you feel more alive than you feel during all of the other days of the year combined. When you spend your time immersed in the elements, your body naturally moves into a state of homeostasis and well-being. When you walk on a beach and let your feet touch the sand, swim in the ocean, and feel the breeze and the warmth of the sunlight on the skin, you are in perfect harmony. We were made to be out in nature.

In the ancient scriptures, the human spine is compared to Mount Meru, *Shiva's* mountain abode in the Himalayas, and the channels of energies that run through the human body are compared to the greatest life-giving rivers of India. This was a way of explaining that everything we see around us exists within us. Remember, the micro-cosmos mirror the macro-cosmos.

Shiva is the "bad boy" god of *yoga.* Who is believed, in Hinduism, to have given the practice of *yoga* to humankind. He is the dreadlock clad, ganja smoking, strong, introverted *yogi,* who hangs out with outcasts and kings alike. He either abides in a state of deep meditation or is furiously performing a dance of creation and destruction. Very similar to how the cycles of nature work.

After you have established a practice to balance your *gunas* and are looking to add more refined practices, you may wish to incorporate another five minutes of any of the *bija mantra* practices below that speak to you.

BALANCING
THE ELEMENTS

EARTH

You know when you need to ground yourself. Connecting with the earth element is a way of establishing a foundation for all practices in *yoga*. Connecting with the earth establishes a sense of grounding, safety, and security. This is especially helpful when you are feeling out of control or in deep emotional discord. Connecting with the force of gravity and letting it hold you will slow you down, bring peace and reset your being. The earth element will gently but firmly ground you back into your own body, so you are stable enough to do more significant, energetic work should you wish to. This element is what most people need because deeply landing in the body will bring the body back into balance.

The poses that balance this element are forward folds, the deep exhalation, and hip openers, which directly stimulate the *muladhara chakra*, the first *chakra* located at the base of the spine and representing the earth element. It is difficult to do any other *yogic* poses without releasing the hips first. Similarly, it is near impossible to find energetic and emotional well-being if you haven't grounded yourself first. Beyond postural *yoga*, we can invoke the earth element through smell. Scents particularly helpful for relaxing into this *chakra* are palo santo, sandalwood, cedarwood, and rosewood smells.

A particularly lovely way to connect with the earth's energy is to walk barefoot in the grass. Smell the grass and lie on it, feeling held by the earth. Let the mother hold you, and surrender into her embrace. This is an excellent way to ground yourself if you need to anchor yourself emotionally or energetically. People who spend most of their time in their heads sometimes experience pain in their feet, or cramping, as if their toes are curling up. This can be an energetic reminder to ground oneself. Find a garden or a park, take your shoes off, and walk barefoot in grass.

Before embarking on any specific *bija mantra* meditation, it's recommended to circulate life force energy throughout the entire subtle body by chanting all the bija mantras: *LAM, VAM, RAM, YAM, HAM, AUM* for eleven rounds. This circulates life force energy and increases awareness of the subtle body, preparing you to focus attention on the center of your choice.

If you want to meditate on earth energy, repeat the seed *mantra LAM* and focus on the center at the base of your spine. Traditionally you would do this 108 times, using a *mala* (a meditation aid with 108 beads) if you desire. I recommend starting with eleven rounds, and if that resonates with you, increase to 108 further down the road.

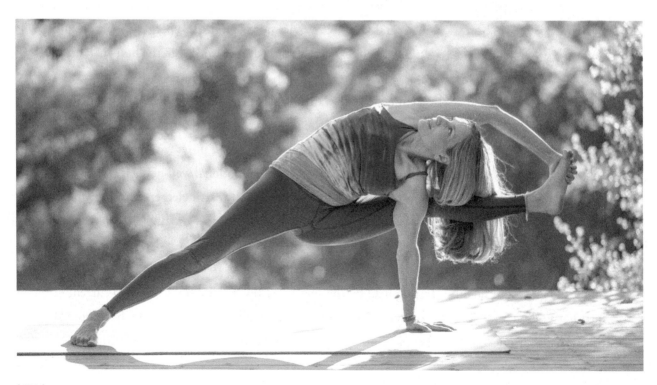

Leila Worby

WATER

Turn to this element when you feel trapped in your emotional body. Neurotic feelings and obsessive, repetitive thinking are prevalent in people with a water imbalance. This imbalance causes the mind to repeat, as if stuck in a loop, and the creative flow stagnates. You also may suffer from self-destructive behaviors, or from anxiety, fear, or frustration. If you experience sexual or reproductive difficulties, you may wish to focus on this center.

As a seasoned *yoga* practitioner, you will eventually be able to tune in to your subtle body, where the elements reside within you, as you move through poses. Usually, you can invoke the water element during transitions between poses. You may experience the sensation of pouring yourself into different shapes. The various prone backbends we do in *yoga* stimulate the *svadhisthana chakra*, which is located three fingers' width below the belly. Consider locust, cobra, and bow poses and spinal waves for developing a relationship with this *chakra*. In Chinese medicine, this point, also known as the *dantian*, located just over the woman's G spot, is considered the seat of our innate power and life force. In *yoga*, this is the creative and reproductive center. It can actually be stimulated from the outside as well as from the inside.

Water is effective in eliminating excessive *rajas*. Taking a cold shower in the morning benefits your physical and emotional well-being by reducing inflammation and toning the vagus nerve. Professional athletes use cryotherapy to repair the body and regenerate the nervous system after intense physical training. If a cold shower sounds more like torture, start with lukewarm showers and decrease the temperature gradually.

Another thing worth trying is to put your wrists, where many meridians run, under ice-cold water. You can also soak your ankles for a while until you get used to the chilly temperature and then enter the water a little at a time until your entire body acclimates. Cold showers make me feel firm and alive, but I prefer them during the warm months of the year because they lower my already-low body temperature a bit too much during the winter months. If you tend to run warm, cold water might be less of a problem for you.

When invoking an element in your practice, you will work on noticing it as you walk through life. Pay attention to how the water feels on your skin during your cold showers in the morning and during cozy warm baths you may indulge in at night. Also, notice the texture and flavor of the water you drink. The sense of taste is directly connected to the water element. Notice the mist in the park during your walk to work. You may also want to submerge yourself in the ocean or simply wet your feet along the shore. Cold plunges are a way of achieving deep communion with this element. You may even want to watch the ocean or a flowing river, for as long as it feels good, while breathing deeply and smoothly. To further commune with the water element, we can bring fountains into our living space to encourage the constant flow of water as it creates tranquility.

There are few things as relaxing and soothing as the sound of flowing water or rain.

The *bija*, or seed, *mantra* for the water element is *VAM*. You may wish to recite this *bija mantra* eleven or even 108 times in meditation as you focus on the energy center located roughly three fingers' width below the belly button.

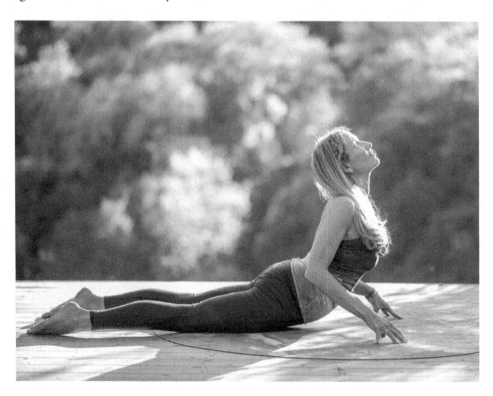

Leila Worby

FIRE

This is the most vital element to invoke when you feel ruled by *tamas* or when you need to boost your energy. Fire will rid you of that constipated feeling of needing to get things moving, both physically and emotionally. Another reason to commune with this element is to boost confidence. The fire element restores our ability to communicate and encourages us to get things done.

As a young woman, I had no one to model confident behavior for me, and it impaired my ability to be successful. I was the first in my family to graduate from college, yet I doubted myself every step of the way. If you doubt yourself, I recommend finding a strong mentor who will take you under their wing, someone after whom you can model your style of communication and your behavior. You may also wish to have a daily meditation practice on the fire element. This will help you develop authentic self-confidence, which is so important for stoking the inner fire throughout life, for it plays an integral role in building a career as well as a social life in your mid-twenties to mid-thirties.

Poses that stoke the fire include any core-engaging pose, from plank to *navasana* (boat pose) and *bakasana* (crow pose). Also, to trigger the fire element within, you can use the deep twists of *yoga*. In the physical body, digestive fire is fundamental to well-being. The deep twists of *yoga* further enhance the immune system by detoxifying internal organs and flushing the lymphatic system.

If you suffer from irritable bowel syndrome (IBS) or a leaky gut, your emotions will suffer as a result. You must take care of these conditions. Physical congestion can cause tantrums in children as well as in adults. My recommendation is to do a *kitchari* cleanse. Eat nothing but *kitchari* for three to five days, three times a day, and your digestive fire will reset. One way to calm the digestive system is a *panchakarma*, or a "five actions" cleanse, at an Ayurvedic clinic to achieve optimal gut health. However, a *kitchari* cleanse is a great place to start. You will find a very basic recipe at the end of the book.

The *pranayama* to stimulate the inner fire is "the breath of fire." Consider how this pranayama resembles the movements of a bellow to stoke the inner fire. That's why it's useful to pacify excessive *tamas*. If you, on the other hand, are trying to pacify *rajas*, you can calm the inner fire by fire gazing. Fire gazing is particularly relevant because the sense connected to the fire element is sight. Light a candle with your morning tea as you do your mediation practice, or repose by the fireplace in the evening. Fire gazing is different from *trataka* on the flame of a candle, which we outlined earlier. Fire gazing will relax and ground you into your body, whereas *trataka* is used to sharpen your focus and alert your senses. Trataka harnesses and focuses the inner fire while firegazing pacifies it.

Fire is used in sacrifice and transformation throughout the history of mankind, fire cleanses and burns through obstacles. The Vikings, as a burial ritual of honor, lit the bodies of great warriors on fire and put them on boats to Valhalla. They believed fire worked as a conductor to usher the souls to the next world. The *bija mantra* for meditating on this element is *RAM*.

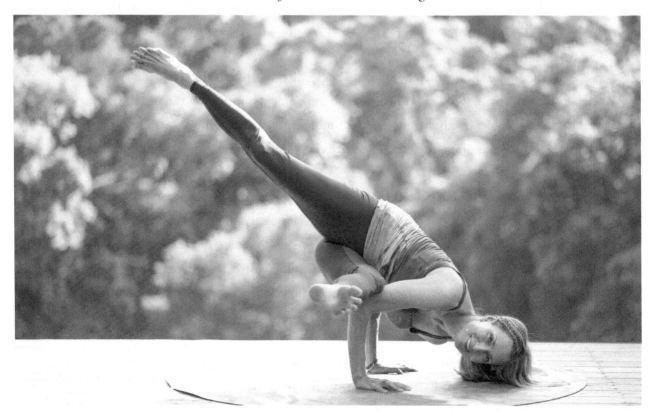

Leila Worby

WIND

The wind element is connected to the heart center, also known as *anahata chakra*. In *yogic* and *tantric* philosophy, this is additionally the true seat of your essence-nature, and is connected to the sense of touch. When a breeze grazes your skin, you may feel as though you've been touched or even caressed by spirit. Energetic, gentle massages, the kind that profoundly touch your subtle body, are perfect illustrations of the connection between the wind element and touch. Touch is a pathway to your subtle body. Massages can work as meditation sessions if you gravitate toward this element. Also, hugging or stroking the cheeks of your loved ones can sooth the subtle body.

When we don't receive enough touch or human connection in our lives, we may benefit from invoking the wind element. We need to connect with other humans more deeply than just on a logical or intellectual level. Often, it's normal to go years without having access to touch, but humans need it to feel balanced and in tune with their emotional needs. I recommend finding a trustworthy, experienced massage therapist to help you recharge the wind element. Another great way to boost the wind element in your life is to take care of a pet that you can cuddle and hold. The energetic subtle body connection between beings doesn't always have to be between humans.

During the lifespan of a romantic relationship, couples usually travel from being completely immersed in each other's energy bodies to being completely separate from each other. And that's often when trouble starts. To reconnect, it can be helpful to do practices together that reconnects the subtle bodies. When you're in love, you're naturally more aware of your subtle bodies, and the will to unite them arises spontaneously. When you've passed that phase, you need to increase your awareness of your subtle bodies before you can unite them again. This doesn't happen by talking to each other, although that also has a place. Doing sensory, engaging activities together can bring you into a state of flow. Some activities include snowboarding, surfing, creating art, attending concerts, or meditating. Find silence together. Focus on sensual, not sexual, touch to recharge the relationship through intentional engagement.

If you are disconnected from the wind element, a deep-seated sense of sadness or depression can take hold of you. In *yoga*, we use the back-bending poses for breathing wind or *prana shakti* (life force) back into our beings. These are poses such as *urdhva dhanurasana* (upward bow), any *rajakapotasana* (king pigeon) variation, and *ustrasana* (camel). If these poses are not available to you, I suggest supported fish pose or the prone backbends recommended for invoking the water element. They will prepare you for these more challenging poses.

Backbends stretch the front of the body and the heart muscle, and they allow us to breathe more fully and take in more oxygen. *BKS Iyengar* recommended backbends to aid depression and soothe pain. Backbends can be likened to a *yogic* kind of CPR that resuscitates the heart that is dying from loneliness and depression. Backbends, in conjunction with "the breath of fire," or *bhastrika pranayama*, can supercharge and stimulate the respiratory system, leaving you feeling energized.

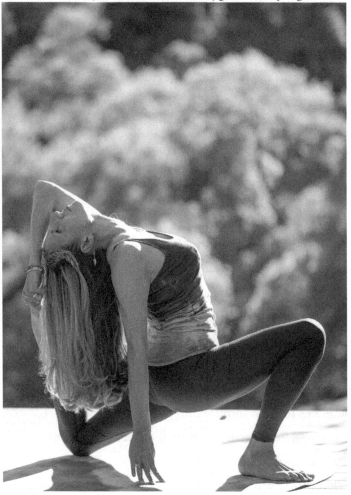

Even if you're not depressed, backbends will have an invigorating effect on your entire nervous system, much like the effect of stimulants such as caffeine, but without the side effects. Other practices that help you stoke the wind are dry brushing the skin and performing *yogic* self-massage, using oil that smells good to you. We usually use sesame oil for this purpose.

The breath is essential when we are focusing on the heart. One powerful practice is to simply pause the breath

Leila Worby

on top of the inhale, for a count of three, focusing on the cave just behind the heart, and then exhaling slowly, deeply, and smoothly.

You may wish to include silent, internal chanting of the *bija mantra HAM* on that pause at the top of the inhale. *HAM* is the *bija mantra* for the heart center. Enjoy this practice for eleven or 108 rounds, if it resonates with you. I personally connect profoundly with this element during my *asana* practice in my garden. The backbends are part of my everyday practice, and when I don't do them, life seems so much duller and grey. To immerse yourself in the elements, I highly recommend doing outdoor practices as often as possible to receive the regenerative powers of nature.

ETHER

This is the all-encompassing container for the other elements. You want to invoke this element if you are looking to find clarity of thought, focused attention, and improved communication skills. This element resides in the three upper *chakras*—the throat (*vishuddhi chakra*), the third eye (*ajna chakra*), and the crown (*sahasrara chakra*). Spirituality resides in the ether. Remember in *yoga*, *dharana*, or focused attention, needs to be mastered before achieving *dhyana*, deep meditation.

The poses that will awaken the throat are poses such as bridge, shoulderstand, plow, and chin stand. The first three will balance your thyroid and endocrine system and are absolutely essential poses for a full, rounded practice. *BKS Iyengar* used to refer to the shoulderstand as "the queen" and headstand as "the king." He cautioned that too much time spent in the headstand would make a person angry. The cooling, calming effects of the shoulderstand are essential for a balanced emotional state.

All the inversions invoke the ether element because they demand focused attention. They are helpful because they pull attention away from your thoughts and produce a state of heightened *dharana*, or focus, that works as an easy segue into meditation. If you've ever been in a space with a group of *yogis* practicing inversions, you may have felt a shift in the atmosphere. This heightened collective focus happens when everyone's brain waves are vibrating on the same wavelength.

If you're not a physical *yoga* practitioner, you can access these upper three *chakras* through meditating on the *bija AUM.* You may also consider chanting or listening to *mantras* and praying. Another option include meditating on the void-by listening to the silence that encompasses and contains all the noises in your surroundings. The sense connected to the ether element is the sense of hearing.

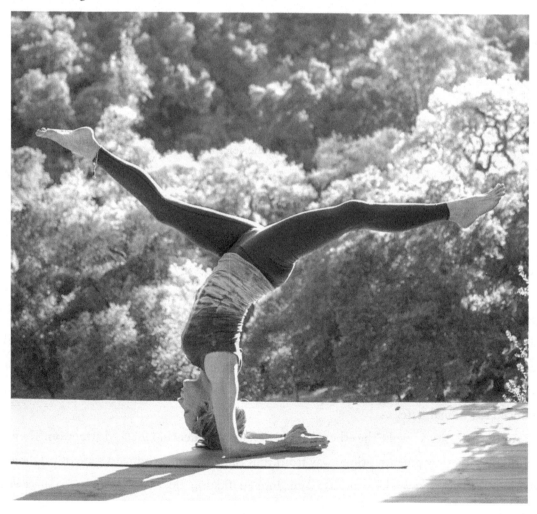

Leila Worby

Growing up in Sweden, I felt melancholy every autumn when the sun set around 3 PM every day for about nine months. The lack of sunlight and warmth was what encouraged me to travel abroad, and it is why I now live in California.

The dark winter months are what prompted the Vikings to travel to more fertile lands, for good reason. It is also why the Viking tradition celebrates the light's return, the peak of light, and fertility so intensely. Light and fertile soil are hard to come by in the northernmost part of the world, so attuning yourself to the solar cycles are particularly important if you reside there.

The sun has always been central to survival. It is responsible for growing crops, warming the body, and providing light to see by. Many *yogic* practices, such as the *namaskars* and the *Gayatri Mantra*, were created as an offering to the sun and, ultimately, as a way of merging with the sun's energy to allow it to circulate inside your subtle body. These practices can give you a lot of comfort during the dark part of the year if you live in the Northern Hemisphere. Doing your practice with the rising sun is particularly useful if you live there.

The sun provides vitamin D, which helps regulate serotonin levels and hormone cycles. Spend fifteen minutes soaking up the sun's rays to achieve optimal well-being. Mindfully eat and drink outdoors on a balcony, in a garden, or in front of a window. Schedule breaks from the computer screen, and take short walks outside throughout the day. Perhaps you can use your lunch hour to walk down to the local park or out in the forest if you have access to one. This time spent in nature will attune you to the rise and fall of the sun and help finetune your endocrine system.

In *yogic* philosophy, the moon is considered the feminine and the sun the masculine force of nature. It's no secret that female hormones run on a monthly schedule just like the moon and some people believe that the male hormonal cycle corresponds to the yearly sun cycle.

To illustrate how everything in nature is perfect in symmetry, the solar cycles work in the same ways as the lunar cycles but on a much longer timespan. Just like the moon waxes and wanes throughout a full monthly lunar cycle, so does the sun and the amount of sunlight we have access to throughout the year. The same cycle is seen in the mechanics of the human breath. Consider the link between the rise and fall of our breath and the rise and fall of the moonlight and sunlight during their respective cycles. Consider further the connection between the fullness, or the pause, at the top of the inhale and the summer solstice—the time of year when the most sunlight is available to us—and how the pause at the bottom of the exhale is similar to the winter solstice, the darkest time of the year. The same link exists between the illumination phases of the moon and the breath, where the fullmoon represents the fullness at the top of the inhale and the new moon the bottom of the exhale.

Once your *yoga* practice becomes a daily ritual, you may begin noticing how cyclical everything in life truly is. You are born, you live a full life, and then your life wanes, and your being eventually returns to earth. Earth nurtures other beings, and so, the life force continues in an endless cycle of creation and destruction.

LUNAR CYCLES

When I attended University in Lund, I worked nights as a nurse's assistant in a ward for psychiatric patients. During full moons, we saw an increase in the number of psychotic people admitted to the hospital. This influx of patients occurred because, during a full moon, energies are elevated. We usually have a lot of energy, but since we're not particularly grounded, we tend to find ourselves extra emotional and sensitive during this time.

In contrast, we often feel depleted of energy and sometimes a bit down on the new moon because of the lack of lunar light. The veil between the spirit world and the human world is considered to be thin during these times. Traditionally, according to *Ashtanga Yoga* philosophy, one should not practice *yoga* during full moon and new moon days because the energies are considered elevated.

As you start adjusting your life to make it more in flow with nature, it's good to craft a new moon and full moon *yoga* practice. It's common to set goals with the new moon. And evaluate and release them on the full moon. In addition I enjoy practicing gratitude on the full moon, because it marks the completion of a cycle, so it's nice to be grateful for everything that has come to fruition but also for the fullness in everything and everyone around us.

The moon mirrors the cycles of our lives. The new moon is reborn, just as it starts to move into a crescent, and it waxes just like the growth of a human walking through life. The full moon symbolizes the peak of human life, and as it starts to wane, so does the life energy in a human, which represents the journey toward death. Death occurs on the dark new moon, and then the cycle starts over again with the next new, crescent moon.

Full moons and new moons are good times for a more elaborate self-care routine because, during these times of the month, energies are heightened and you want to do what you can to soothe yourself. For most people, performing a long self-care practice every day is not sustainable, but investing in self-care once or twice a month is often sustainable. You might add the grounding practice of dry-brushing your skin, followed by oiling your entire body, before your candlelit bath, if it speaks to you. My skin gets dry during the winter months, so I like to oil myself after the bath without rinsing the oil off my body. The key is to find a monthly ritual that is sustainable in your life. Do not create demands. Instead, create enjoyable rituals that enhance your life experience.

SOLSTICES AND EQUINOXES

I recommend doing some form of contemplation on the solstices and equinoxes. Because they mark transition points between the seasons. It's nice to take a moment to consider what the season that just ended brought in terms of growth and visualize what you want to call in before the upcoming season. And it further attunes you to the seasons and the flow of nature. The spring equinox is a good time to do detoxifying *yoga* practices, such as deep twists and inversions, in preparation for summer. Eat light, raw fruit and vegetables, and polish the body by dry-brushing and oiling the skin. We usually feel like practicing *yoga* more playfully, stronger, and longer during the spring and summer months when we have access to a lot of sunlight, which invigorates the physical body. The autumn equinox presents a good opportunity to prepare for mental productivity with practices that move our attention inward again, where creativity can be sparked. Autumn and winter are seasons for creative, cerebral endeavors, physical rest and restoration, and ingestion of hearty, warming stews. Slow flows, yin and restorative *yoga* practices are conducive to these junctions of the year.

Honor the solar cycles by creating a ritual around these very powerful junctures. A great tradition to begin might be to spend the summer solstice out in nature, camping and practicing *yoga* with your close friends. Perhaps rent a cabin for skiing, *yoga*, and fire gazing in the mountains during the winter solstice. Let your intention setting and releasing span the whole year instead of monthly as you would do during the new and full moon.

As outlined earlier, a wonderful *mantra* at this time of year is *Asatoma Sadgamaya*. Find it on Spotify to get the rhythm down. I like to do *yoga* to the sound of a *mantra*, and once I get the rhythm and words down, I chant them.

Sun cycles affect physical energy levels more than they affect the emotional body, whereas the moon greatly affects the emotional body. To understand this, think about how sunlight affects your physical body. The times of year when we are exposed to more sunlight make us feel like moving our body more, and we have energy to be active, productive and radiating. Versus when there is little sunlight available, which makes us feel like hibernating. The moon, on the other hand, impacts the emotional sheet of the body. When the moon is full it tends to bring us into a heightened state of awareness that triggers our primal instincts. The moon is connected to our intuition and inner world and the Lunar energy is good to use when you need to seek counsel from and connect with your intuition. Lunar energy is also very conducive to meditation and any spiritual practices. While solar energy will help you accomplish things in the world and heal your physical body.

Close to the summer solstice, I love sunset practices. It's like a celebration of the abundance of sunlight at this time of year. Write down whatever you wish to release for the year. Burn it and give it to the wind near the ocean or any body of water.

The winter solstice occurs at the bottom of the exhale. It marks the darkest day of the year, when the sun starts gracing us with its warmth and light more and more in the upcoming waxing

Leila Worby

cycle. It's considered a rebirth of the sun in some traditions. It's a good time for intention setting. The best time to do so is at sunrise. This is a powerful time of day at this time of the year, because you want to harvest the grace of the sun's light as much as you can now, due to its scarcity at this time of year. Massage and oiling of the body are great for this time of year to promote circulation and warmth. It's a good idea to hike in nature and do yin and restorative postural practices and meditations that guide your attention internally. When you set your intentions and goals, they are for the upcoming year this time, not the month. If you have a mind that thrives on structure, you can make your monthly intentions feed into your yearly goals and then reevaluate them and release what no longer serves you during the summer solstice. This is a great time to practice inward listening and deep meditation.

CREATING A SANCTUARY IN YOUR HOME

Always start with creating a space in your home that you ideally only use for *yoga* practice. If you can't find such a space, roll out your mat facing east, if possible. I like to light a few candles and dim the light slightly. I also enjoy burning some incense. If it resonates with you, you can have all the elements represented in your surroundings. Perhaps you would like to create a small altar on which to place a cup of water or a small fountain to invoke the water element. Some crystals can be used to represent earth; a lit candle represents fire; and incense represents air and ether.

Many people like to decorate their altars with pictures of enlightened beings because it's taught in *yoga* that the pictures evoke and transmit the energy of those beings. Possibilities include *Christ*, *Krishna*, *Amma* and *Yogananda*. If symbols are more effective for you when invoking a state of reverence and peace, place a cross or a *yantra* on your altar. If creating a dedicated space in this way is too much of an effort in the beginning, don't do it. The most important thing is that you practice. Your body is already a temple.

Smelling essential oils attunes you more to your senses and your connection with nature as well. And it can work as a real treat to take in the smells of lavender, sandalwood, and rose. You may wish to explore using a humidifier to enjoy them for longer amounts of time in your home. To further commune with nature, you can bring it indoors with you. Bring your favorite plants to your desk, buy flowers regularly for no reason. They are beautiful, and they encourage you to acknowledge the beauty and perfect symmetry that exists in nature. I love honoring the solar and lunar cycles by placing tree branches in my home and decorating them with the current season's ornaments. This provides me with a sense of peace as I am reminded of the cyclical nature of life.

CHAPTER 5

The *Namaskars* and Poses

NAMASKARS

Namaskars, or salutations, were initially offered as a ritual of greeting and reverence for the sun and the moon. They are lovely to practice at sunrise and sunset. They provide a vehicle for moving into deep communion with solar and lunar energies. Let the salutations circulate the life force throughout your being and connect you to the powerful energies of the sun and the moon. *BKS Iyengar* said that his body was a temple and the *asanas* (poses) his prayers. This is exactly the reverence with which we should approach our movement meditation.

On a physical, bodily level, the *namaskars* are all we need for a full practice. *Namaskars* circulate the breath, strengthen and open the body, and create space in all the critical places. Stronger *namaskars* are a full-body workout on their own. What makes them superior to any other workout is that they are a moving mediation and they connect the breath with the body's movement. If you adopt light *ujjayi pranayama* as you move through your *namaskar*, you will notice yourself moving deep into your own being. If you are a mover with a busy mind and lots of physical energy, this will be the best practice for you.

The *namaskars* are repetitive, so they allow your body to open up more and more as you continue to flow through them. These days there are many trendy new *yoga* practices offered online. While having easy access to *yoga* can be a wonderful opportunity, unfortunately, many of these trendy practices have omitted the *namaskars*. The repetitiveness of the *namaskars* doesn't seem to resonate with the attention span of modern practitioners, so many practitioners are robbed of the meditative benefits the *namaskars* provide. I urge you to explore the *namaskars* in your own practice with patience and diligence. Tradition usually only survives for centuries because it has powerful effects. Before discarding it and playfully reinventing the wheel, I would urge you to at least let it become part of your practice for a while, so that you can judge its impact for yourself.

CLASSICAL NAMASKAR*
(SATTVA PROMOTING)

Come to standing. Bring your feet together and press down gently, through the four corners of your feet. Keep your spine straight. Start with your palms together, in front of your heart center (thumbs against your sternum).

Take a few deep, slow breaths here. On your next inhale, keeping the palms together, raise your arms overhead. Perhaps add in a bit of a backbend (Think up and over), if that feels good to your body. Exhale as you fold forward and bring your palms to the earth, touching the ground, if that's comfortable for you. Bend your knees as much as you need to make this happen.

Inhale and come halfway up, placing your fingertips to your shins as you look out and up, past the front of your mat, and broaden your collarbones by keeping your shoulders lowered, squeezing your spine (rather than raising or hunching them). Exhale, lowering your hands, one on each side of your right foot, and step back with your left foot, drop the left knee to the earth, and curl the toes under.

Inhale, ballooning your chest open, as you send your sternum forward and up. Pull your shoulder blades down and back, keeping them away from your ears. Gaze to the sky. Exhale, grounding down through your palms, and step your right foot back into downward-facing dog.

Take one deep, full breath here, letting the energy pour through your palms and the soles of your feet. Then, flow forward into a high plank on the inhale. Slowly lower down to the ground, either by bringing your knees, chest, and chin to the earth or by lowering through chaturanga dandasana (yogic pushup). Whatever feels best for you will work.

If you did knees-chest-chin, rise up through cobra. If you did chaturanga, rise up through an upward-facing dog. Exhale as you flow back to downward-facing dog. Inhale, and step your left foot forward into a low lunge. Exhale.

Inhale, and step the right foot to meet the left. Come halfway up, fingertips to shins. Exhale as you fold forward. Inhale, and roll up vertebrae by vertebrae, all the way to standing, as you raise your arms up and over your head. Palms together, draw your hands to your heart center, gently pressing the thumbs to your sternum. This is one round. Continue in this way for fifteen minutes, or about ten rounds. Some people enjoy flowing through namaskars while listening to their favorite mantras, and this can also be a good way to keep track of time.

* I recommend silently or internally chanting the *bija mantras* of the *chakras* as you move through this *namaskar*. This will circulate the life force even further and leave you energized. The *bija mantras* for the different poses in the *namaskar* are listed together with their respective pictures.

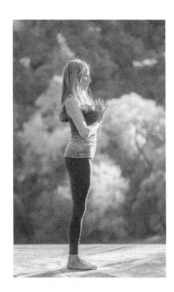

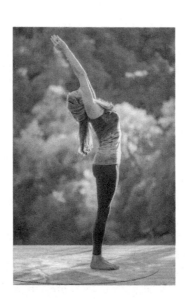

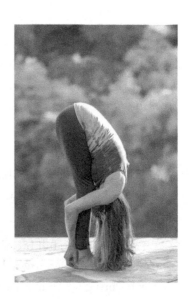

1. Aum Hram   2. Aum Hreem   3. Aum Hroom

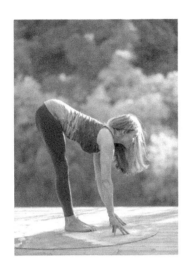

4.

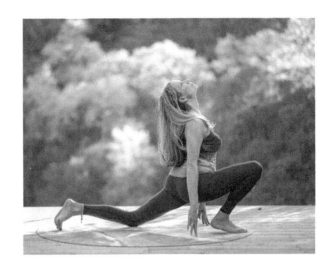

5. Aum Hraim

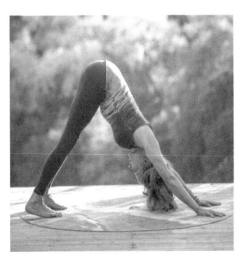

6. Aum Hraum

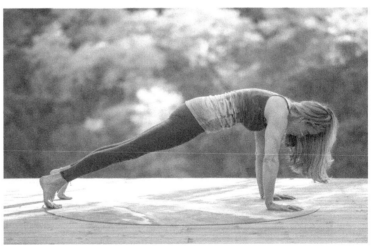

7.

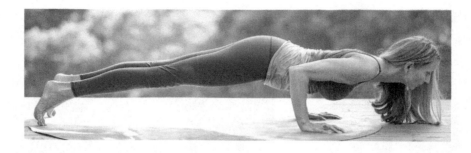

8. Aum Hrah

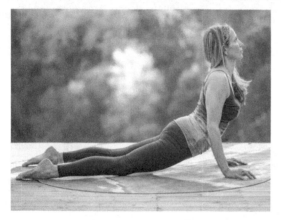

9. Aum Hram

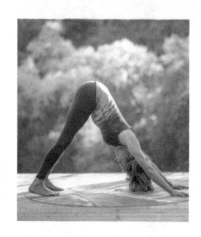

10. Aum Hreem

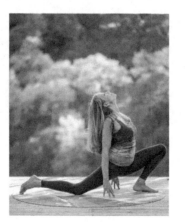

11. Aum Hroom

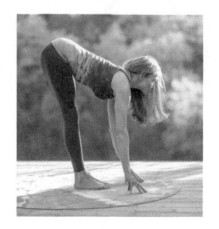

12.

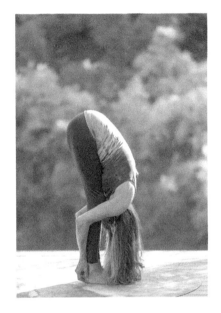

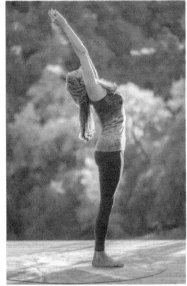

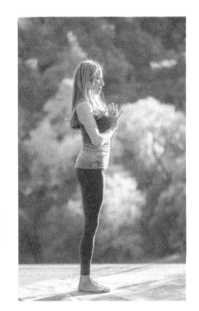

| 13. Aum Hraim | 14. Aum Hraum | 15. Aum Hrah |

CHANDRA NAMASKAR (RAJAS PACIFYING)

Chandra namaskar allows you to move into deep resonance with the calming, relaxing, and cooling lunar energies that most people need in today's fast-paced world. This is a refocusing meditative movement inward, toward unity with your own inner essence. Treat it with utmost reverence.

Begin by standing with your feet together or hip-distance apart. Place hands in prayer at your heart center. Inhale as you raise your arms overhead, balloon your chest open, and send your heart center up and perhaps even back in a small backbend. Really allow the expressions of this namaskar to unfold. Do not go to your most profound depth immediately. Exhale as you fold forward, and touch the earth with your hands, bending the knees as much as you need to.

Inhale and come halfway up. Exhale, step the right foot back, and drop the right knee to the ground, so that it's resting in a low lunge. Uncurl the toes if that feels good. Inhale and lift your hands and arms to the sky.

Stay with a vertical spine, or arch your back as much as feels good, keeping the core engaged. Don't drop the head entirely. Maintain an energetic connection between your chin and your chest. Step back to a high plank position, and lower your knees, chest, and chin to the earth. Send your sternum forward and up as you rise into low or high cobra.

On an exhale, lead with your lower belly as you flow back to downward-facing dog. Inhale and step the right foot forward. Then, lower the left knee to the ground, so that it's resting on the ground in a low lunge, and uncurl the toes if it feels good. Let your arms float up over your head, and reach your hands to the sky. Exhale as you step your left foot forward, coming halfway up. Then, fold deeply.

Inhale as you rise all the way up to standing and reach up. Exhale as you bring the hands to prayer at your heart. Repeat these movements several times, for a set of fifteen minutes. Alternate which foot you step back with as you let yourself move into meditation.

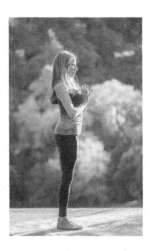
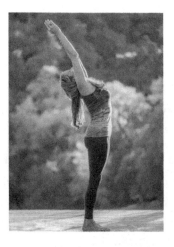
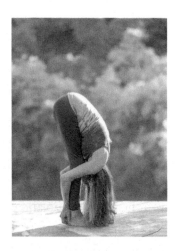

1.   2.   3.

Leila Worby

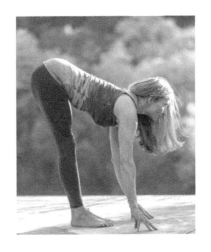

4.

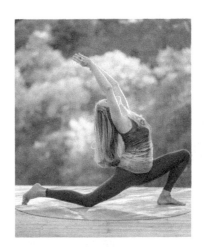

5.

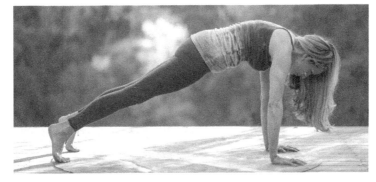

6.

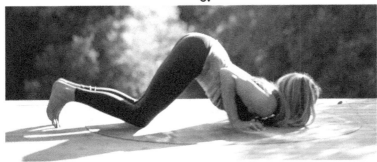

7.

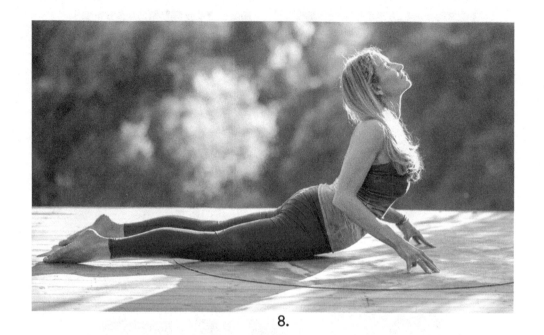

8.

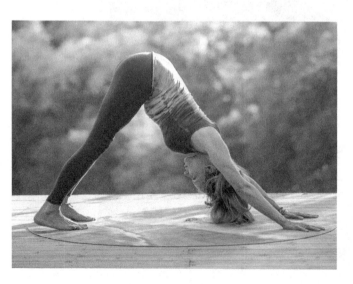

9.

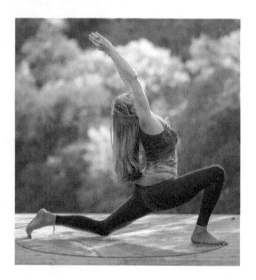

10.

Leila Worby

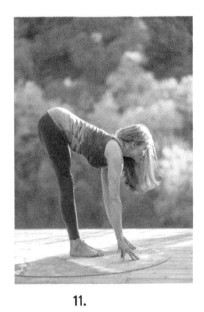

11.

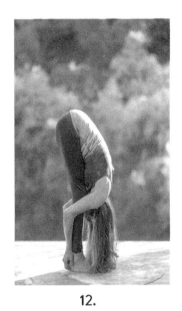

12.

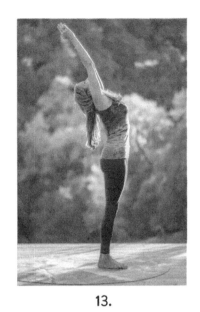

13.

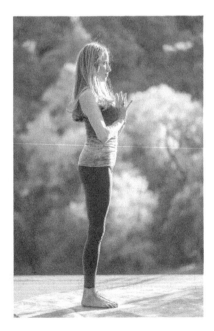

14.

Surya Namaskars A and B
(*Tamas* Pacifying)

I recommend three rounds of *surya namaskar* A, and three to five rounds of *surya namaskar* B. *Surya* means "sun" in Sanskrit. It is the most energizing *namaskar*, and it will stoke the life force in you. This *namaskar* is a contemporary take on the classical *namaskar* and has greatly impacted modern *yoga*. It has incredible benefits on the physical body.

SURYA NAMASKARA A*

Stand with your feet together, big toes touching, hands in prayer at your heart center. Inhale, and raise your arms overhead, palms together. Exhale, hinge from the waist, and fold forward to touch the earth, bending your knees as much as you need to protect the lower back. Step or jump back to high plank. If you jump, try to land in chaturanga. If you step back to high plank, slowly bend your elbows, letting them grace your ribcage. If this is hard, do it with your knees on the earth, you may need to lower all the way down to the ground. Hover for a few breaths in the pose's final expression, and then use your toes to push yourself forward into upward-facing dog. Roll the shoulders back and down your spine. Exhale back into downward-facing dog. Take three breaths here, step or jump your feet to meet your hands, and come halfway up. Exhale and fold. Inhale, and rise all the way up. Exhale, and bring your hands back to your heart.

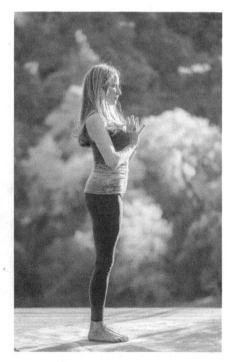

1.

Leila Worby

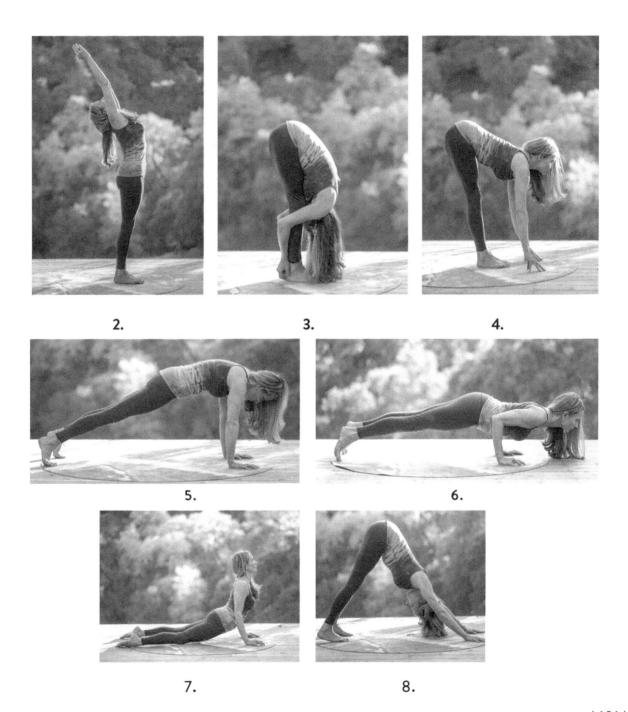

2.

3.

4.

5.

6.

7.

8.

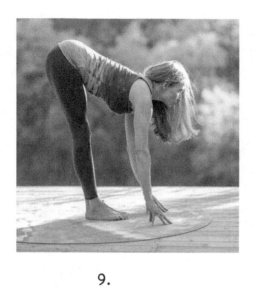

9.

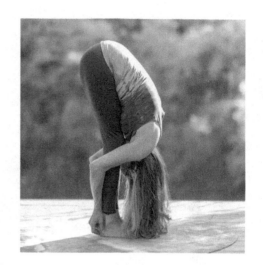

10.

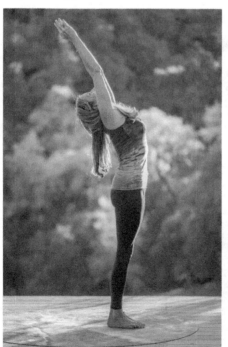

11.

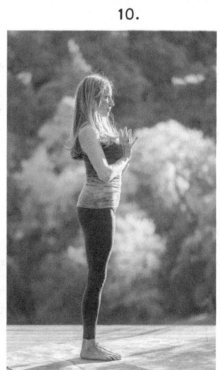

12.

Leila Worby

Begin in *samasthiti*, which is Sanskrit for "stand upright." Move hands to prayer at the heart center. Move the feet together, big toes touching. Exhale as you bend your knees, letting your fingertips graze the mat. Inhale, and sit down in an imaginary chair, letting your arms rise up over your head, palms together and toes lifted. Exhale and fold forward.

Inhale, and come halfway up, broadening through the chest. Exhale and either jump back to *chaturanga dandasana*, or step back into high plank with the toes tucked under. If you step back to high plank, slowly bend your elbows, letting them grace your ribcage for *chaturanga dandasana*. If this is hard, do it with your knees on the earth and ankles crossed. Hover for a few breaths (it may be more comfortable to lower all the way down to the earth instead of hovering), and then you use your toes to push yourself forward into an upward-facing dog. Roll the shoulders back and down your spine. Exhale and return to downward-facing dog.

Take a breath, and on your next exhale, step the right foot forward. Inhale, and rise up into warrior one. Warrior one is a deep lunge with the back foot rooted into the earth, toes of the back foot pointing forward at a 45-60 degree angle. Try to square your hips toward the front of the mat. This is the goal, but it's not anatomically possible for most practitioners. Move toward that energetic movement as long as it feels good. Don't force the angle or shape. Just enjoy the stretch. Exhale, and draw the hands to the earth, stepping the right foot back into a high plank. Slowly lower into *chaturanga*. Inhale, and slowly rise into upward-facing dog. Exhale back to downward-facing dog. Inhale, and step forward with the left foot. Root into the outer edge of your back (right) foot, and press into the front (left) foot as you rise to warrior one over your front left foot. Raise the arms overhead and bring the hands into prayer. Roll the shoulders back and down your spine. Now, draw your hands to the earth and step back to a high plank. Flow from *chaturanga* to upward-facing dog, and then to downward-facing dog. This is a resting rather than active downward-facing dog. The difference is that, in the resting version, we take a pause and collect our breath and we get comfortable in the pose, inhabiting it with a sense of steadiness and ease. In an active downward-facing dog we might do spinal waves, calf stretches, side body stretches, or we might raise a leg to the sky to exert more energy.

Take three to five breaths here, and when ready, either step or jump your feet to meet your hands. Come halfway up. Exhale and fold. Inhale as you bend your knees, letting your fingers touch the earth. Then, rise up into chair pose. Straighten your legs, and come back to *samasthiti*, with your hands in prayer at the heart center.

* If you need to keep your feet hip-distance apart or your hands wide as you reach your arms overhead in chair pose, or warrior one, do so. The *namaskars* are outlined here as they were taught traditionally. As you adjust and improve, move toward the traditional expression for a more nuanced practice.

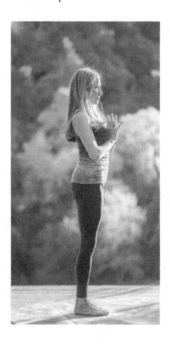

1.

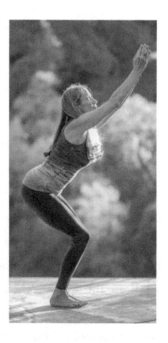

2.

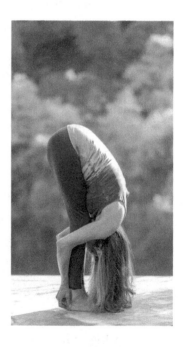

3.

Leila Worby

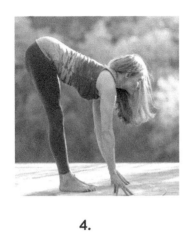

4.

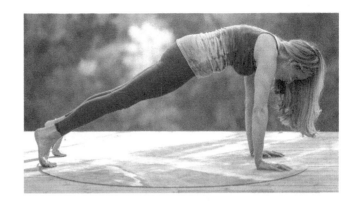

5.

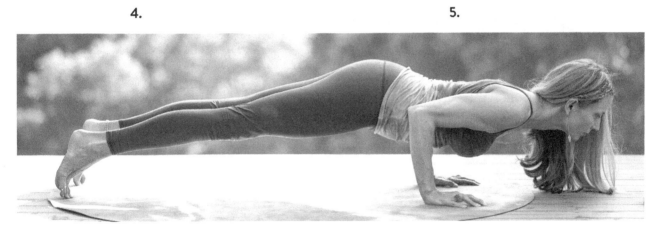

6.

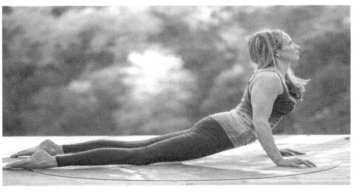

7.

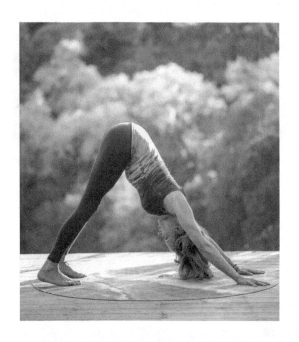

8.

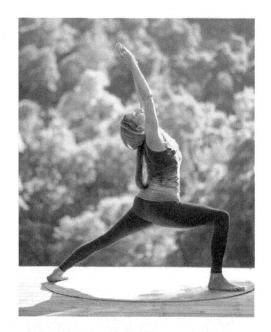

9.

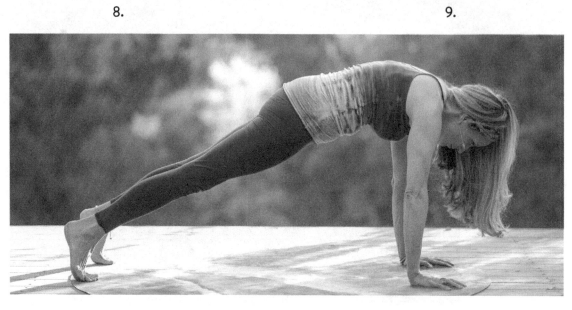

10.

Leila Worby

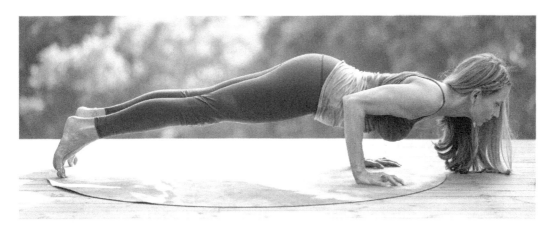

11.

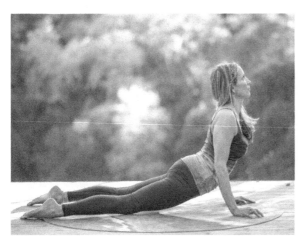

12.

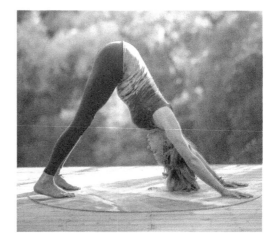

13.

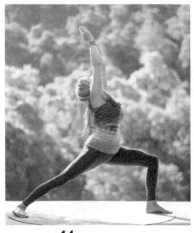

14.

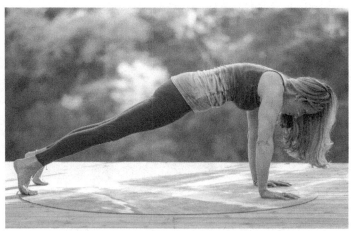

15.

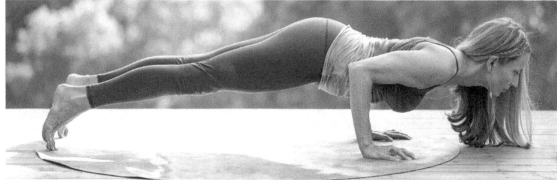

16.

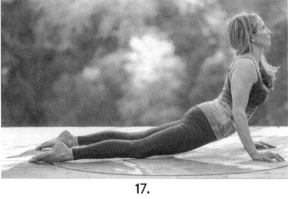

17.

Leila Worby

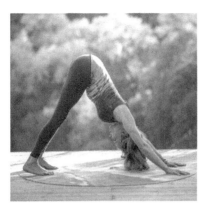

18.

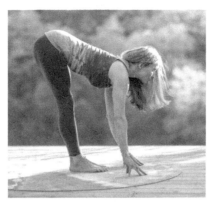

19.

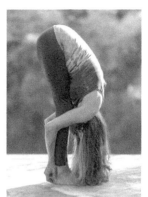

20.

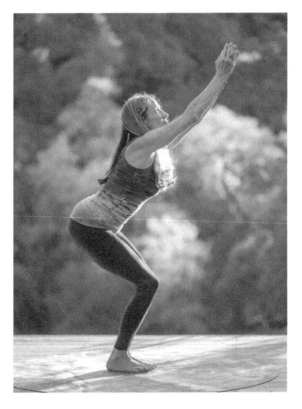

21.

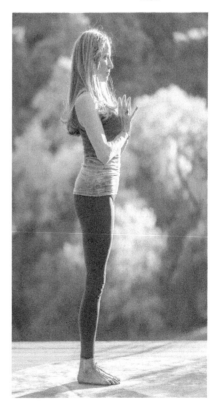

22.

THE POSES

The poses of *yoga* have an almost magnetizing effect on practitioners. They immediately grab your attention, and make you want to defy gravity and levitate through the *vinyasas* (movement between poses) in the same way the *yogis* filled with *prana*, or life force, do. The poses and the movements have an almost magical pull. According to Pattabhi Jois, the founder of *Ashtanga Yoga*, the more lifetimes you've lived as a *yogi*, the stronger this pull is.

In traditional *Yoga* we start by circulating the energy through the subtle body as we move through the *namaskars*. We then slow down and "take a seat" in the poses, using energetic movement and the breath to awaken the *chakras* (energetic vortexes or wheels along the spine). Incidentally, *asana* (pose) means to take a seat. The poses belong to different families that stimulate different *chakras*, and every family shares the same energetic expression. They start out as small expressions and end in full expressions of life force as the body opens more with practice. In this chapter you will find an overview of the families of poses, along with the *chakra* and element that they invoke. To stimulate the life force and encourage it to rise up through our subtle body, we begin with stimulating the root, or earth, *chakra* and work all the way up to the crown *chakra* in terms of how we sequence the poses. First, we gently stimulate the root *chakra* through the seated forward folds and the hip openers. Then, we invoke the water element through prone backbends that increase in intensity. From there we stimulate the fire element through core engaging practices and twists. At the end of our practice we are prepared to enter the back-bending sequence that stimulates the wind element and the heart *chakra*. The closing poses are all intended to allow you to enter the most subtle of the elements—the ether. These poses stimulate our three spiritual centers, the *vishuddhi* (throat), the *ajna* (third eye) and the (*sahasrara*) crown.

If you have ever studied the *Ashtanga Yoga* series, you will see how the same idea is played out on a larger scale. The first series is all about the forward folds and hip openers and focusing on establishing a strong base. The second series moves the energy up to the heart center, and the

Leila Worby

poses of the third series takes you to the ethereal realm, with poses that help you take flight and that continue to move the energy from the heart to the throat, then to the third eye and the crown and beyond. We see this thoughtful sequencing mapped out in most styles of traditional *yoga* and going deep into at least one traditional *yogic* lineage will help you learn how to properly feed your entire energy body. "*Hatha*" means "force," and it refers to forcing the physical body, or more specifically, churning the spine. It also refers to the forcing of the breath through *pranayama*, in order to build and raise life force energy.

During your own practice, try to move your intention inward and notice your body and breath as you move through the poses. Remind yourself that breath carries *prana*, or life force, so the deeper and slower you breathe, the more you are permeating your being with life force. You want to spend three deep, slow *ujjayi* breaths in every pose. Only go as far into each pose as feels good, and keep your breath smooth, deep, and even. Let your breath be your guide as you explore the poses. Let them open and unfold over time. If you're in restorative poses, you may wish to spend two to five minutes in each pose to allow your body to relax into the deeper benefits of the poses.

There is always a point in your body where your attention rests in every pose or transition of *yoga*. Attaining the perfect stretch for your body is what makes poses so meditative. You want to cultivate a razor-like focus where your attention rests as you move into the pose. Like life in general, *yoga* happens just as much in the transitions as in the stillness of the poses themselves, so be equally as mindful as you enter and exit the poses as when you're in them. Work on making the transitions between the poses as calm, slow, and matched with your breath as possible. That's where you will find flow. This is the practice. This is movement mediation. *Yoga* is about unity with your true inner essence. It's an intimate, private practice best explored in solitude or with a teacher.

Forward Folds and Hip Openers (Earth)

CHILD'S POSE—*BALASANA*

Sit on your heels and reach your arms forward. Flow forward and rest your torso on your thighs, and your forehead and arms on the earth. Keep hands in prayer or clasped, with the index fingers extended. Keep your glutes as close to your heels as possible, maybe even resting the glutes on tops of the heels. Keep the gaze down and inward.

Benefits: This is a grounding pose that gently opens the hips, instills profound relaxation, and induces *pratyahara* (a withdrawal of the senses). Child's pose stimulates the muladhara center, which governs your safety and security, your foundation.

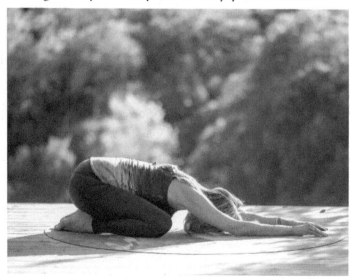

Leila Worby

SEATED FORWARD FOLD—*PASCHIMOTTANASANA*

From a seated position with the sitz bones rooted into the earth, extend the legs forward. The upper torso folds forward at the crease of the hips, keeping the spine long. Broaden through the collarbone and keep the gaze forward. You may use a strap or a belt around the balls of your feet or keep your legs bent to make it easier to maintain a flat spine.

Benefits: This is a grounding hamstring stretching pose. It lubricates and creates space between the vertebrae of the spine and profoundly relaxes you and promotes *pratyahara*, withdrawal of senses.

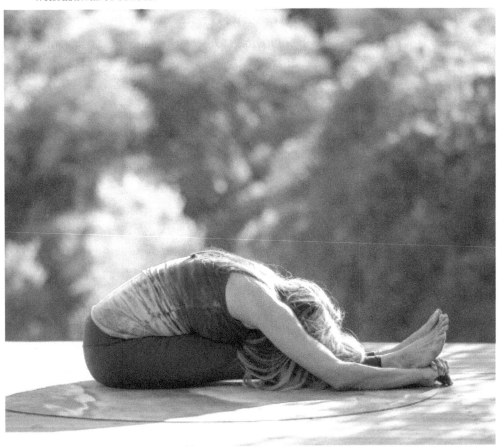

HEAD TO KNEE POSE—*JANU SIRSASANA*

Sit on the floor with your legs straight in front of you. Bend one knee and place the sole of your foot against the inner part of your opposite thigh. Your extended leg and knee should be comfortably pressed onto the floor, and your bent knee will have an outer, upper rotation. Center your chest and belly over your extended leg. Grow your spine long. Then, fold over your straight leg, walking your hands out in front of you. Keep a long spine, reach for your ankle or toes with your hands, or rest your arms alongside your extended leg. You may wish to use a strap for this pose.

Benefits: This is a hip opening hamstring stretch that creates space between the vertebrae of the spine. This pose stimulates the *muladhara chakra*, the root and earth center that is our foundation. This pose also facilitates *pratyahara*, the withdrawal of the senses.

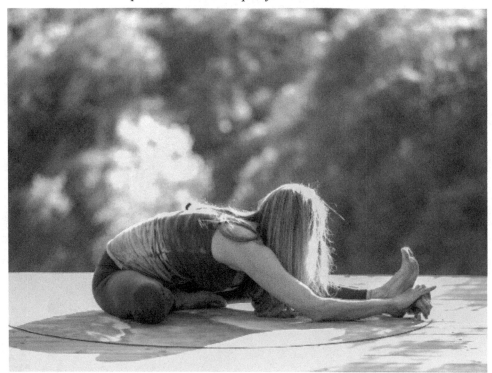

Leila Worby

ONE LEG FOLDED FORWARD BEND—TRIANGA MUKAIKAPADA PASCHIMOTTANASANA

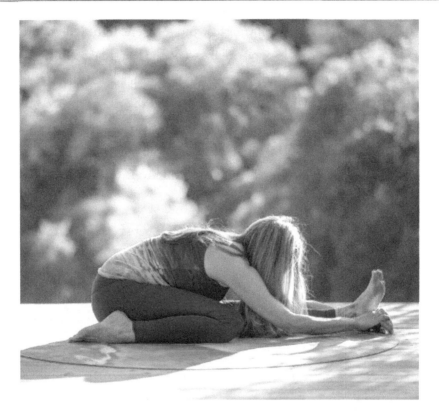

Sit back on your heels, the tops of the feet touching the mat. Shift to the side as you release your left leg in front of you. The right leg remains bent, and the top of the right foot rests on the earth, next to your right hip. Slowly start reaching forward, letting your sternum lead the way. Perhaps you can hold on to your ankle or maybe even your toes. Please listen to your ankles and your knees in this pose, and go only as far as feels good.

Benefits: This stretches the quads, hamstrings, hip flexors, and the ankles, while promoting relaxation. It stimulates the *svadhisthana chakra* (center of reproductivity and creativity) and the *muladhara* (root) *chakra*.

HERO'S POSE—*VIRASANA*

From a kneeling position on the floor (with a folded blanket to pad your knees, shins, and feet if necessary), sit with your glutes between your feet and rest here. If the glutes don't comfortably rest on the floor, raise them onto a block placed between the feet. Make sure both sitz bones are evenly supported. Leave a thumb's width between the inner heels and the outer hips. Rest the hands on the stomach, lap, or thighs. Lift the back ribs and the top of the sternum. Widen the collarbones as you release the shoulder blades away from the ears. Lengthen the tailbone into the floor to anchor the back torso. Only if you can sit comfortably between your feet without support, lower your back onto the floor. Stretch your arms over your head and clasp the elbows. Maintain a straight spine as you enter and exit this pose.

Benefits: This pose stretches the quads and creates space between the vertebrae of the spine. This pose stimulates the *muladhara chakra*, the root and earth center that is our foundation. It also stimulates the *svadhisthana chakra*, our reproductive and creative center. This pose additionally facilitates *pratyahara*, the withdrawal of the senses.

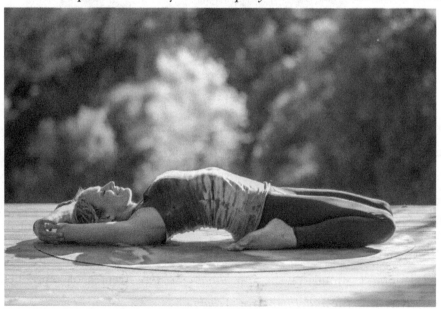

Leila Worby

BOUND ANGLE POSE—*BADDHA KONASANA*

In a seated cross legged position, bring the soles of the feet together. Then bring the heels as close to the groin as possible, keeping the knees close to the ground. With your hands holding the tops of your feet, open your feet like a book, pulling the tops of the feet toward the earth and soles toward the sky. Fold forward. The shoulders should be pulled together and down and the spine straight.

Benefits: This is a wonderful hip-opening pose. *Baddha Konasana* promotes fertility and balances the reproductive system. This is a great pose to support women struggling with hormonal imbalances and during pregnancy. It stimulates both the *muladhara* (root) and *svadhisthana* (reproductive) *chakra*.

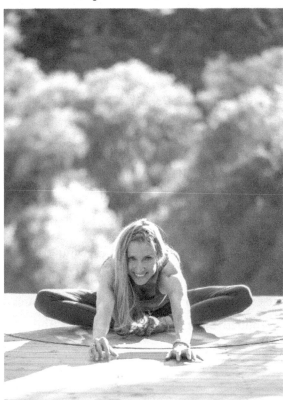

WIDE-LEGGED SEATED FORWARD FOLD—*UPAVISTA KONASANA*

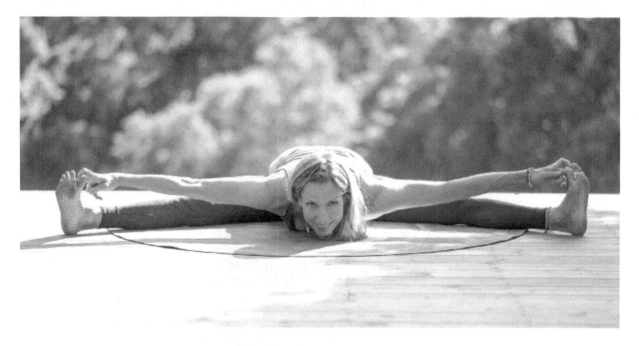

Sit on the earth with your legs stretched out in front of you. Open your legs wide to the sides. Place your hands behind you, keeping the fingers pointing away from you. Gently use your hands to push yourself to the front part of your sitz bones. Fold forward for five deep breaths, reaching forward with your heart, and working to keep the spine as straight as possible.

Benefits: This pose promotes relaxation, aids digestion, and stretches the hips, abductors, hamstrings, and calves. It creates space in your spine and gently massages the kidneys and, as such, aids with detoxifying the body. It stimulates the *muladhara* (root), *svadhisthana* (reproductive), *manipura* (solar plexus), and *ajna* (third eye) *chakras.*

Leila Worby

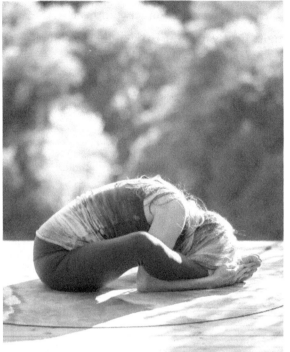

Seated on the earth, ground through your sitz bones, and open your legs a little wider than the hips. Then, bring the soles of your feet together. Let the knees point out to the sides. Fold forward and thread your arms between the legs, wrapping your arms under your inner calfs and over your shins, eventually holding on to the tops of the feet. Rest your head on the inside edges of your feet or on a block or a pillow (placed on the ground between your feet or under your heels). You may take full *kurmasana* if it speaks to you. Do so by bringing your shoulders under your knees. Keep your arms, with the palms toward the earth, stretched out to the sides. Then, drop your chest to the ground as you straighten the legs, radiating through the balls of the feet.

Benefits: This is a hip opener, hamstring stretch, and shoulder stretch (if you move into the full version). It promotes deep relaxation and stimulates the *muladhara* (root) *chakra*, which is your sense of security and foundation. It profoundly triggers a withdrawal of the senses (*pratyahara).*

Squat down by bending your knees, and rest your glutes on your calves with toes pointing forward or out to the sides. You may need to roll up a blanket and place it under your heels in the beginning. Bring your elbows to the insides of your thighs, gently pressing to open them as much as feels right.

Benefits: *Malasana* stretches the thighs, groin, hips, ankles, and torso. It tones the abdominal muscles and aids with elimination. It increases blood flow in the pelvic area and balances sexual energy. It improves balance, concentration, and focus. *Malasana* stimulates the *svadhisthana chakra*, the creative and reproductive center, and the *muladhara* (root) *chakra*, your sense of security and foundation.

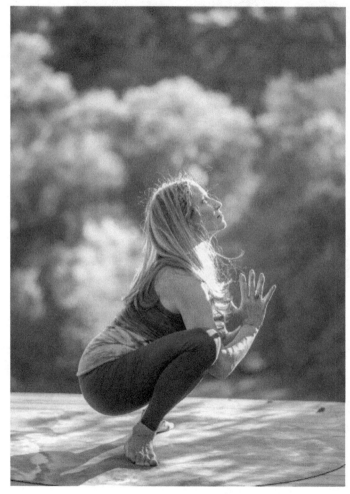

Core Twists and Arm Balances
(Fire)

BOAT POSE—*NAVASANA*

From a seated position, legs straight out in front of you, lift one or both legs up. Angle the thighs about 45-50 degrees, relative to the earth. Keep the legs straight and your body resembling the letter V, or a boat. The tailbone is lengthened and grounded into the earth. Spread the shoulder blades across the back, and reach the hands straight forward so the arms are parallel to the earth. Tip the chin slightly toward the sternum so that the base of the skull lifts away from the back of the neck. Gaze forward.

Benefits: *Navasana* engages and stabilizes your core, and it intensifies the digestive fire that resides in the *manipura* (navel) *chakra*. It also strengthens your hip flexors.

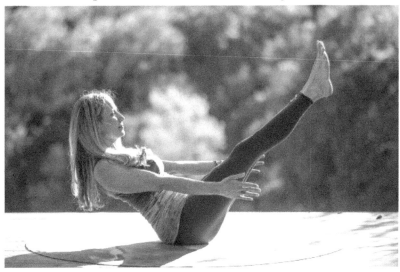

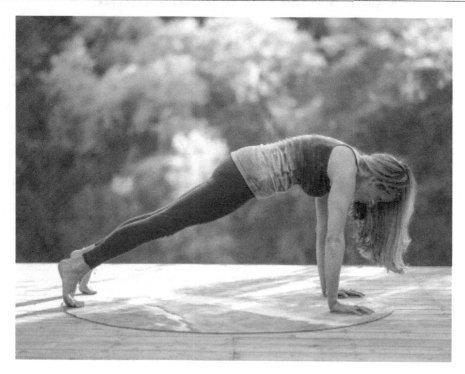

Start on your hands and knees, curl your toes under and send your hips up, so there is a strong line from your crown to your midsection and your heels. Strongly press into your hands so that your upper body rounds. Try to broaden through your heart and chest, while maintaining the straight line from crown to heels. Be mindful to engage your core so that you don't let your hips or your midsection sink too low.

Benefits: This pose works the core, creating stamina and strength. It aids digestion and stimulates the *manipura* (fire and solar plexus) and *ajna* (third eye) *chakras*.

Leila Worby

FOUR-LIMBED STAFF POSE—*CHATURANGA DANDASANA*

From a high plank, push yourself forward while bending your elbows to a 90-degree angle. Your elbows are pulled into our ribcage like wings to help stabilize you. Keep your line strong throughout your body. Radiate your strength through your crown and your heels. If this is too difficult for you, try dropping your knees to the earth while crossing your ankles. Flow forward from there. You may also wish to lower all the way to the ground and omit the hovering that takes place between this transition and upward-facing dog.

Benefits: This tones and strengthens the entire body, especially your core and your shoulders. It requires a lot of wrist flexibility. Four-limbed staff pose stimulates the *manipura* (confidence and fire) center.

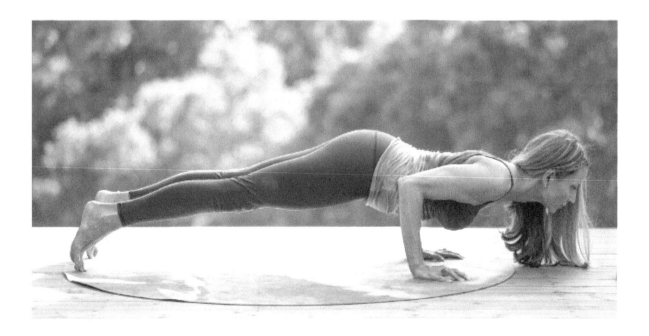

SEATED TWIST (EASY)—*PARIVRTTA SUKHASANA*

Come to a comfortable seated, cross-legged position. Keep your spine straight. Place your right hand with the fingers pointed away from you at the base of your sacrum as support. Place your left hand on your right knee. Take a deep breath and on the exhale, root your sitz bones deeply into the earth and start twisting toward the right, doing your best to look over your right shoulder. Inhale and slowly move back to center.

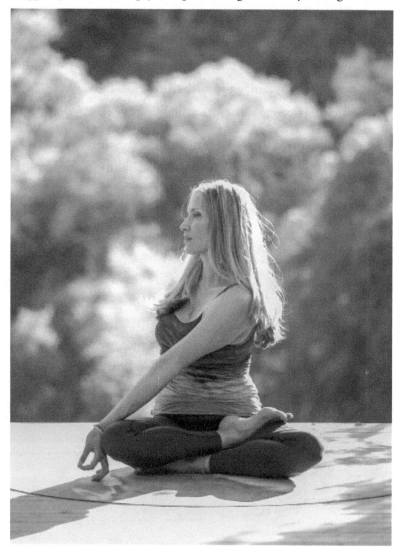

Benefits: This drains the deep lymph nodes and aids digestion and the immune system. It keeps the spine supple, preparing it for deeper backbends. It moves the energy from the *muladhara* (root) to the *sahasrara* (crown) and stimulates the *anahata* (heart) center.

Leila Worby

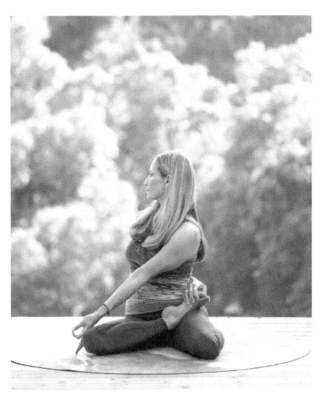

Start in a seated position. Bend your right knee so the top of your shin and the foot are facing the earth. Bring the left foot to the inside of the right thigh or on top of it in *ardha padmasana*. Ground down into your sitz bones, maintaining the spine straight and then start twisting. Place your right hand on the left knee. Perhaps bind by wrapping your left arm around the back of your waist and gently grasping the top of the left foot with the left hand. Inhale as you let the spine rise, and exhale to twist.

Benefits: This pose is hip-opening and quad-stretching. It aids digestion and drains the deep lymph nodes. It keeps the spine supple, preparing it for deeper backbends. It moves the energy from the *muladhara* (root) to the *sahasrara* (crown) and stimulates the *anahata* (heart) center. The seated twist also promotes trust in yourself and a connection to your inner animus or anima (in Jungian psychology, the masculine part of your personality if you're a woman and the feminine part if you're a man). In *yogic* terms we refer to this as the inner *Shiva* or *Shakti*. Binding positions in which you hold yourself by wrapping the limbs promotes this connection to the other side of your persona for an integrated experience of true unity.

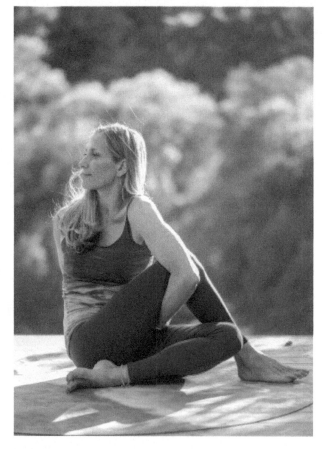

Sitting with legs stretched out in front of you, bend the left leg and bring the left foot next to your right hip, with the outside of the leg and foot resting against the earth as much as possible. Bend your right leg, place the right sole of your foot on the outside of your left leg, toes in line with the left knee or in front of it. To achieve the twist, support your sacrum by placing your right hand there, fingers pointing away. Then hook your left elbow over your right knee. Pull yourself in close. Hug yourself. Straighten your spine. On an exhale, begin to ground down through the sitz bones and twist toward the right. If possible, move the left elbow to the outside of the right knee. Then, place your left hand on top of the left foot. Alternatively, you may wish to thread your left arm through your right leg and grab the fingers of the left hand with your right hand. Twist on the exhale.

Benefits: This pose aids digestion, drains the deep lymph nodes in support of the immune system. It keeps the spine supple, preparing it for deeper backbends. It moves the energy from the *muladhara* (root) to the *sahasrara* (crown) and stimulates the *anahata* (heart) center.

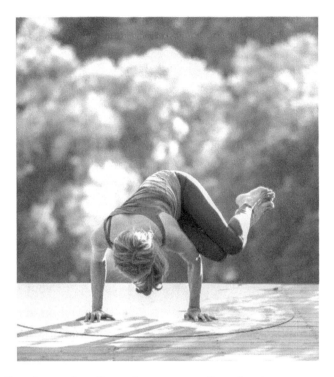

Come onto the balls of your feet from the most profound twist you can muster in a revolved chair. Try to bring your right elbow to the outside of your right hip and your left elbow to just above the outside of your right knee if you are twisting to the right. Bring your hands to the earth, shoulder-width apart. Fingertips should face the long side of your mat. Lean forward into your fingertips, try to align your shoulders just above them. Shift your weight to your hands and hover.

* This and the rest of the armbalaces listed below may not be accessible to you yet.

Benefits: This pose strengthens the shoulders and the core, and it promotes balance and focus, aids digestion, drains the deep lymph nodes to support the immune system, and keeps the spine supple. It moves the energy from the *muladhara* (root) to the *sahasrara* (crown) and stimulates the *anahata* (heart) center to promote bliss, self-confidence, and clarity of mind. The act of balancing further stimulates the *ajna* (third eye) *chakra*.

CROW POSE—*BAKASANA*

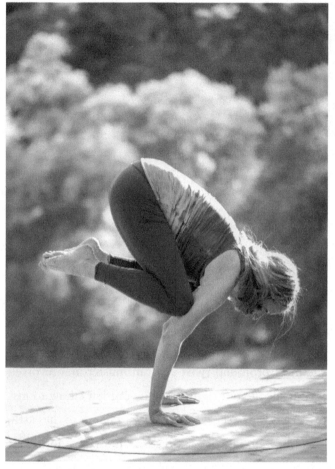

From a deep squat on the balls of your feet, toes turned out slightly, place your hands on the earth, shoulder-width apart, just in front of your feet. Round your upper back and broaden through your chest as you lift your glutes into the air, and then walk your feet closer to your body until you can press your knees into your armpits. Transfer your weight into your hands, pressing your fingertips and the four corners of your hands into the earth. The weight is in the fingertips. Release your right foot from the earth, and then the left, finding your center of gravity. Move into a hovering position, balancing on your hands. Keep your gaze on the mat. If it is difficult to find the shelf under your armpits, you may place the knees lower, on the top of the outsides of your triceps. Then, engage your inner thighs to squeeze your arms, lift one foot at a time and hover.

Benefits: This is a hip-opening and core-engaging pose that requires a lot of wrist flexibility. The fire of the *manipura chakra* (solar plexus center) is strong in this pose. *Manipura* governs self-confidence and assertiveness. The act of balancing further stimulates the *ajna chakra* and cultivates both the inner fire and digestive fire.

Leila Worby

FIREFLY POSE—*TITTIBASANA*

From a *yogic* squat come up on the balls of your feet and move your shoulders under your knees and hamstrings. Sit down as you press into your palms and radiate your legs, one at a time, out to the sides. This is a fun arm balance that lifts your spirit.

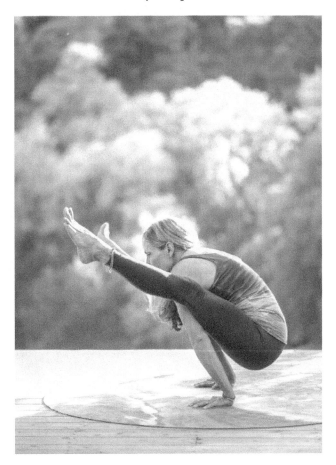

Benefits: This pose opens the hips and engages the core. It requires flexible hamstrings, strong wrists, open hips, and a strong core. In this pose, the energy moves from the *muladhara* (earth) *chakra*, to the *manipura* (fire) *chakra*, and lastly to the *ajna* (third eye) *chakra*.

SIDE PLANK—VASISTHASANA

From a high plank, release your right hand and extend your right arm to the sky. At the same time, stack your right foot on top of your left foot. Send your side waist to the sky.

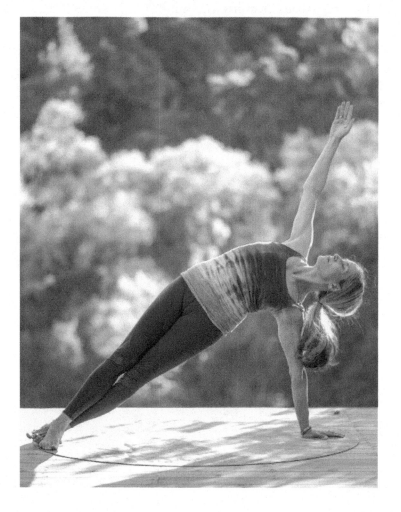

Benefits: This pose strengthens and tones the side waist and the wrists but simultaneously requires a lot from them as you are resting your entire weight on just one wrist. It stimulates the *svadhisthana* (reproductive) center and the *manipura* (fire and confidence) center.

Leila Worby

I recommend using a wall to prevent yourself from falling into the backbend. Usually, if you can hold a plank without a problem, you are able to hold a handstand. The easiest way is to come into downward-facing dog and kick one leg up and over, drawing the other knee into your chest as a lever. Aim to get your hips up and over your shoulders. Alternatively, you may also jump into a

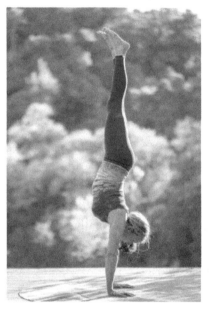

tuck position by bending your knees in a downward-facing dog, jumping like a frog, and drawing both knees to your chest. This is usually easier for people with limited hamstring flexibility. Move the hips up, hover just above the shoulders, and extend both legs up. Another option is to come to a downward-facing dog with your butt against the wall and walk your feet up the wall until your body is in a pike position, forming the letter L. From here you may wish to extend one leg to the sky and after having figured out the hip placement, perhaps both legs. Give it time and practice, and it will come. Think about your fingertips and the mounds of your palms as being in constant negotiation when it comes to actually holding your handstand for longer amounts of time.

* Please skip this pose if it doesn't resonate with you, or if you feel too weak to hold yourself in a handstand. Skip it if you have problems with your wrists, shoulders, neck, or elbows or if you have glaucoma or high blood pressure. This goes for all the inversions. Please always listen carefully to your body.

Benefits: Handstands drain the lymphatic system and engage and strengthen the core, the shoulders, and the wrists. They promote balance and focus. In terms of energetic centers, handstands stimulate the *manipura* (fire) center and the *ajna* (third eye) center. They bring you into the immediate moment and promote self-confidence and razor-like focus.

Backbends (Water and Wind)

CAT/COW POSE—MARJARYASANA/BITILASANA

From a tabletop, take a deep breath. As you exhale, press into your palms, and drop the crown of your head toward the earth. Round your upper spine, broaden through the chest, and tuck your tailbone. You want to feel your navel glued to your spine. This is Cat. From here, inhale slowly and smoothly as you look ahead of you, melting your stomach down and sending your tailbone to the sky. This is Cow. Continue flowing between these poses on the breath as long as it feels good, noticing every vertebra of the spine.

Benefits: These poses awaken the spine and the life force. They further release tension along the spine, stretch the shoulders, and release the neck. It is a wonderful movement for cultivating connection between movement and breath. It additionally stimulates *svadhisthana*, the center that governs creativity and reproductivity.

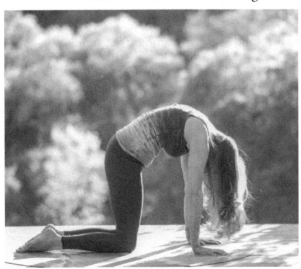 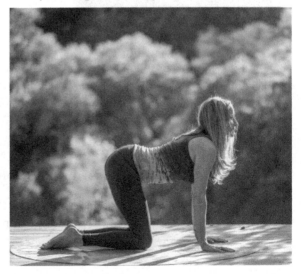

Leila Worby

BALANCING TABLE—UTTITHA MARJARYASANA

Starting from a tabletop, with your shoulders over your wrists and your knees under your hips, step the right foot back, and slowly press the heel toward the sky. Then, reach the left arm out in front of you. The gaze is on the thumb.

Benefits: This is a great balancing pose that promotes coordination. It's also core-engaging and stabilizing. It opens the chest and maintains a supple spine. It stimulates the *ajna* (third eye), *anahata* (heart), and *manipura* (solar plexus) *chakras*.

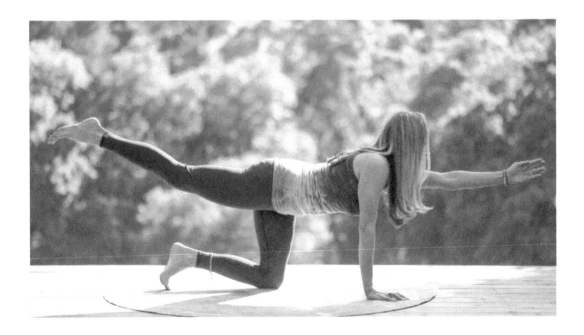

From a tabletop, lower the chest and chin toward the earth. Your fingertips are aligned with your shoulders. Gently hug your ribcage with your elbows, and place the majority of your weight in the hands. Your legs are bent and your toes are curled under.

Benefits: This increases the flexibility of the neck and shoulders while opening the chest. *Ashtanga pranam* also strengthens the shoulders and the legs. It uses the force of gravity to stimulate the throat center or *vishuddhi chakra*, as this center rests toward the earth. It's your center for speaking your truth.

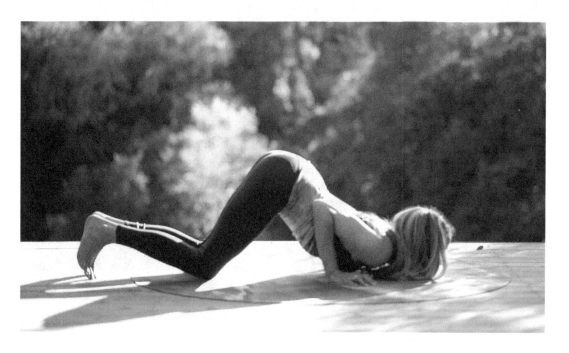

Leila Worby

UPWARD-FACING DOG—*URDHVA MUKHA SVANASANA*

Most commonly you will enter this pose from *chaturanga dandasana*. With your toes curled under, push yourself forward, sending your sternum forward and up. Your weight is in your hands, and they are positioned under your shoulders. Your shoulders are hugging your spine and pulled down toward the ground. Your pelvis and thighs are hovering just over the earth. Your legs are activated and strong.

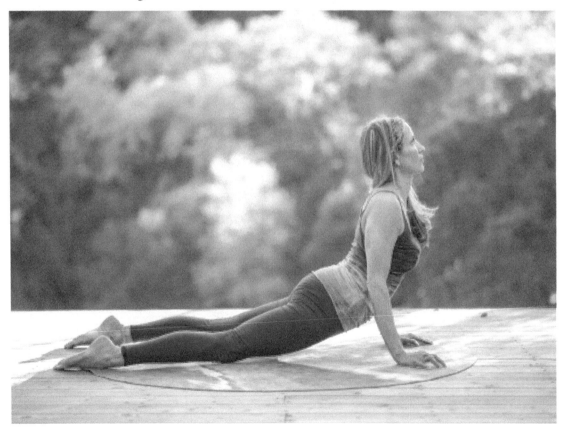

Benefits: This maintains the supple spine and builds strength in the shoulders and legs. *Anahata* (heart) and *manipura* (solar plexus) *chakras* are stimulated through this pose.

From a high plank, send your hips back and up so that your body resembles an inverted V. Root down firmly through the palms, fingers spread wide. You want your wrist creases to align with the top of your mat. Press your heels toward the earth, and draw your rib cage toward the tops of your thighs. Don't worry if you need to bend your legs in order to make this movement happen. You want to feel your belly button sticking to your spine in this pose.

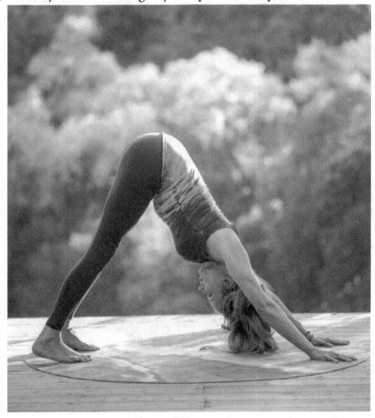

Benefits: This pose stretches your shoulders, hamstrings and ankles. It strengthens your wrists and shoulders. Downward-facing dog calms your mind, stimulates your digestion, and builds your stamina. This pose stimulates the *svadhisthana* (reproductive) *chakra* and the *anahata* (heart) *chakra*.

Leila Worby

LOCUST POSE—*SHALABHASANA*

From a prone position, lying on the belly, with the arms alongside the body, palms facing up, lift the legs away from the floor until you are resting on the lower ribs, abdomen, and front pelvis. Firm your glutes and extend through strong legs and active, pointed, toes. Raise the arms and shoulders, keeping them parallel to the floor with active, straight, fingers. You may wish to clasp the hands behind the hips, if that is comfortable for you. Gaze forward or slightly upward, being careful not to force the chin up and crunch the back of the neck. Keep the base of the skull lifted and the back of the neck long.

Benefits: This pose strengthens the lower back, hamstrings, and glutes. It opens the chest and stimulates the *anahata* (heart) *chakra* and *svadhisthana* (reproductive) *chakra*.

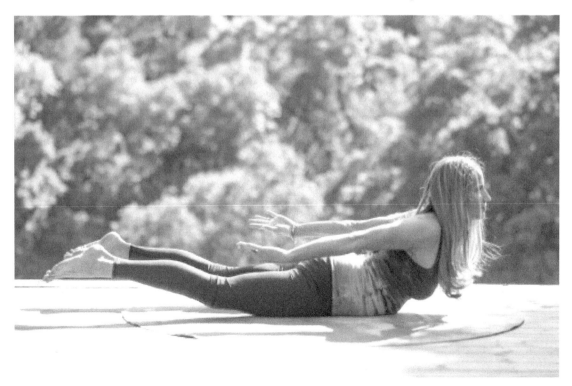

HALF FROG POSE—ARDA BHEKASANA

Lying on your belly (resting on your forearms, elbows under your shoulders, as in sphinx pose), position your left arm in front of you, parallel with the short edge of your mat. Bend your right leg, grab the foot with your right hand, and press the foot toward your right hip/glute as you press into your left forearm. To deepen the stretch, pivot the fingers of the right hand so they point toward you.

Benefits: This pose provides quadricep, hip flexor, and shoulder stretches as well as a small backbend. It stimulates the *anahata* (heart) *chakras* as well as *svadhisthana* (your creative and reproductive center).

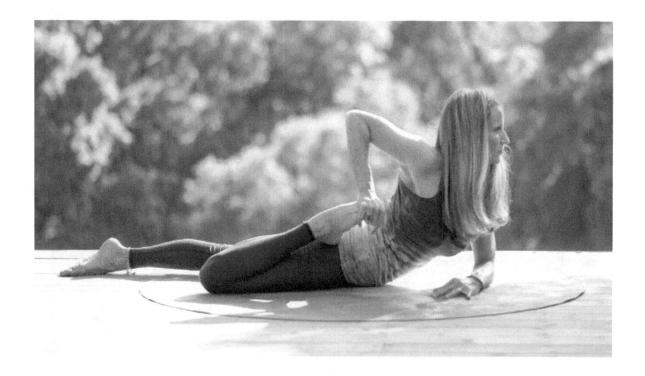

Leila Worby

COBRA POSE—BHUJANGASANA

Start by lying on your belly. Bring your feet together so the big toes touch. Rotate your thighs inward. Pull yourself forward on your elbows, creating space between the vertebrae. Rest here for a few breaths. Place your hands on the earth, press into your pinky toes, and pull the shoulder blades together and down your spine. Lift your chest without placing any weight in your palms, using just the strength of your lower back. This is a low cobra.

If it feels good, you may press into your palms and rise slowly to a high cobra. The movement should come mainly from using the strength in the lower back. Avoid pressing too strongly into your palms without awareness of the lower back since this will only compress the vertebrae in the lower back and create injury. Please listen to your lower back, and make sure you pull your shoulder blades down your spine. This pose requires substantial spinal flexibility. Be wise enough to listen deeply to your body and stay at the place that's just right for you.

Benefits: This pose maintains a supple spine and strong lower back. It stimulates the *svadhisthana* (creative and reproductive) center, opens the *anahata* (heart) center, and allows you to breathe fully.

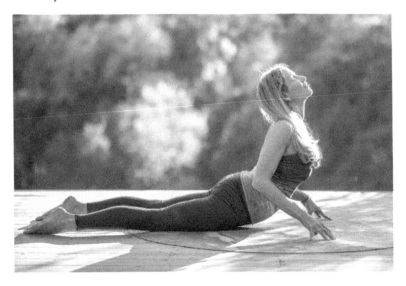

BOW POSE—DHANURASANA

From a prone position with the abdomen on the earth, grab your ankles with your hands (but not the tops of the feet). Keep the knees no wider than the width of your hips. Lift your heels away from the buttocks. At the same time, lift your thighs away from the earth, working opposing forces as the heart center, hips, and back open. The gaze is forward and up. To deepen, move your gaze and the balls of your feet toward the sky.

Benefits: This gently opens the chest without requiring too much of your shoulders or wrists. It's also a nice shoulder stretch. Listen to your lower back as you slowly rise into your bow pose. There should never be pain in backbends. If that happens slowly come out and work in locust pose instead. Bow pose stimulates the *anahata* (heart) center as well as the *svadhisthana* (creative and reproductive center). It's an expression of compassionate, embodied love.

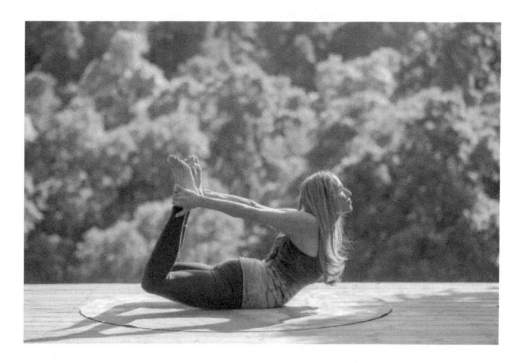

Leila Worby

CAMEL POSE—*USTRASANA*

Enter camel pose from a kneeling position with the knees hip-width apart and thighs perpendicular to the earth. Rotate the inner thighs slightly inward with the glutes engaged but not hardened. Tuck the tailbone under. Support your sacrum with your fingertips (fingers pointing upward). Gently push your sacrum forward while opening your chest by pulling the shoulder blades together and down the spine. Send your sternum up and back for a few breaths, working to create length in the spine while slowly ballooning the chest open. Slowly lower one hand at a time so the palms are on top of the heels, fingers pointing toward the toes. Keep a connection between the chin and the chest for a few breaths before you drop the head back slowly as far as is comfortable to you. You may wish to skip this step altogether. Breathe here for five deep breaths.

Benefits: Camel require open hip flexors and a flexible neck and spine to feel comfortable. I strongly recommend starting by placing your hands on blocks that you may place just outside your feet on the earth. This will allow you to rest your attention in your heart center while you're in the pose by bringing the earth closer to you. You don't want a pinch in the lower back distracting you or the sensation of discomfort in your neck. You want to cultivate an energetic connection between your chin and your chest. If you drop the head back before your body is ready for it you may hurt your neck. You may also cradle the crown of your head with your hand, keeping the elbow aligned with the crown of your head, to support your neck. Camel is a lovely pose that allows you to breathe fully. It stimulates the *anahata* (heart) *chakra*, which is a center of pure, selfless love, compassion, and bliss.

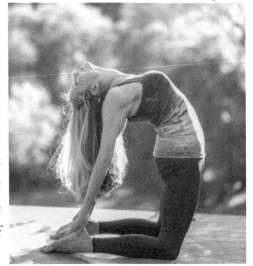

REVERSE TABLE POSE—ARDHA PURVOTTANASANA

If the upward bow is too challenging for you, this pose is a good alternative. Sit on the earth with your legs stretched out in front of you. Bend your knees and place your feet hip-distance apart, a foot or two away from your tailbone. Root your hands just behind your hips, palms down, fingers pointed toward your feet. Inhale and press into your feet and your hands. Send the hips up and spread the sternum wide, relaxing the neck. The gaze is toward the sky or your nose. Your body now resembles a table.

Benefits: This strengthens the glutes and the wrists, and it opens the chest and gently stretches the spine. It stimulates the endocrine and respiratory systems as well as the *vishuddhi* (throat) *chakra*, *sahasrara* (crown) *chakra*, and *ajna* (third eye) *chakra*.

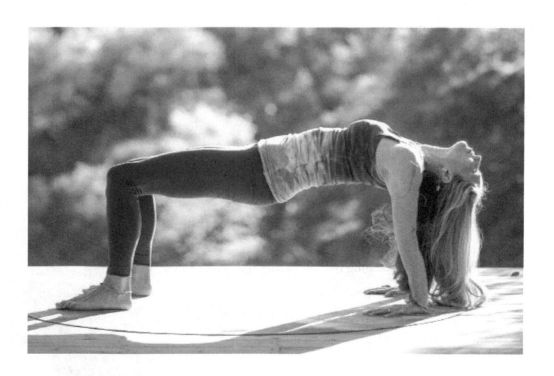

Leila Worby

BRIDGE POSE—SETHU BANDHA SARVANGASANA

From a supine position, on your back, bend your knees and place your feet hip-distance apart. Press into the four corners of the feet as you press the hips up. Roll your shoulders under your chest, and reach your hands toward your heels, clasping your hands and interlacing the fingers. The thighs are parallel to the earth as you lift your ribcage and open the heart. The back of the neck rests on the earth. The gaze is to the sky.

Benefits: This is a chest-opening and thyroid-balancing pose as well as a lovely shoulder stretch. This pose stimulates the *vishuddhi* (throat) *chakra*, the center of clear communication, truth, and self-expression.

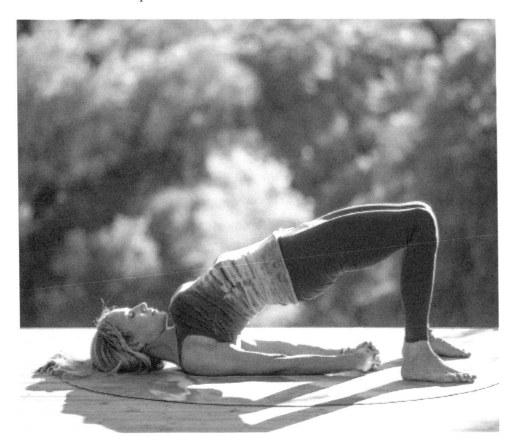

UPWARD BOW POSE—URDHVA DHANURASANA*

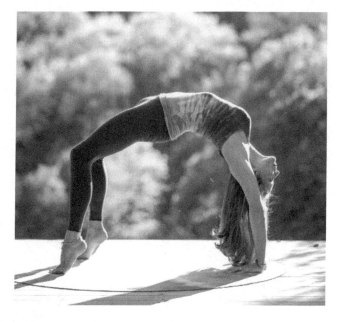

From a supine position on your back, bend your knees and place your feet quite far away from your tailbone—if your arms are by your sides you want your feet just by the fingertips to start out. Place your hands by your ears, palms facing the mat, so that your fingers are pointing toward your shoulders. Then press into the ground as equally with your feet as with your hands and start rising slowly, sending the hips up. Weight is equally distributed into the hands and feet. It may be helpful to rise onto the balls of your feet. Move your shoulders toward your wrists by pressing into your feet, this will open the torso and create space in the lower back. Keep your glutes lightly engaged. To come down, slowly lower vertebrae by vertebrae. You may consider doing this pose three times. Please move slowly as you enjoy deeper backbends, it's important to let your spine open. Too often I see students exploding into backbends, try moving in slow motion and place your inner gaze at your heart center. Should you start feeling discomfort or even pain in another part of your body such as your lower back, wrists or shoulders, stop and slowly move out of the pose.

* Only attempt this pose if you have strong, healthy shoulders, spine, and wrists.

Benefits: This pose keeps your spine supple, stretches the shoulders, and strengthens the wrists. It opens the chest and allows you to breathe fully. This pose is suggested to ease depression. It moves the energy from the *muladhara* (root) *chakra* to the *sahasrara* (crown) *chakra* and stimulates the *anahata* (heart) *chakra* profoundly.

Closing Sequence (Ether)

SHOULDERSTAND—SALAMBA SARVANGASANA*

From a supine position, engage your abdominals to raise the hips straight up toward the sky while

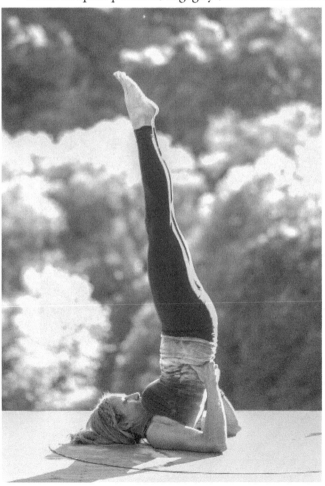

supporting the lower back with your hands. The legs are fully extended, and the toes are active. Let the upper back, shoulders, and triceps rest on the earth. Keep the elbows shoulder-width apart. Your forearms are off the earth, and the torso is perpendicular to the earth. The neck is flat on the earth, and the chin is tucked. The gaze is inward.

* Only practice shoulderstand if it's appropriate for your body (in particular, your neck).

Benefits: This pose stretches the neck and strengthens the core and glutes. It stimulates the thyroid and endocrine systems and promotes fertility and relaxation. Shoulderstand stimulates the *vishuddhi* (throat) *chakra* and helps you move inward and to speak your truth.

PLOW POSE—HALASANA*

From the shoulderstand pose, slowly bring your legs over your head so the toes touch the earth. Keep the legs engaged, and clasp the hands behind the back. To exit, bring the hands back to your hips for support, engage the abdominals, and return to a shoulderstand before lying in a supine position, on your back.

* Please only practice Plow if you have a healthy neck and a strong, healthy spine.

Benefits: This stimulates the thyroid and deeply stretches the spine and neck. The *vishuddhi chakra* is stimulated here, your center for communication and speaking your truth.

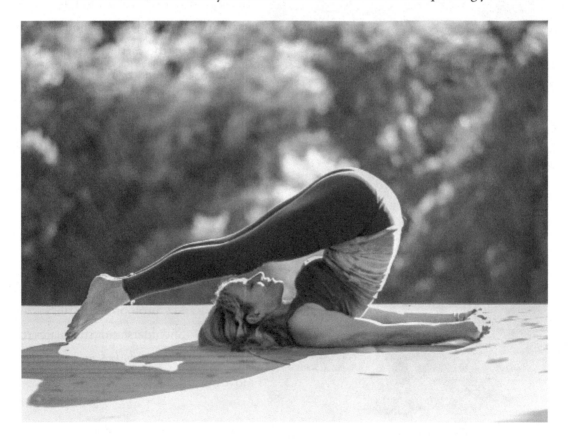

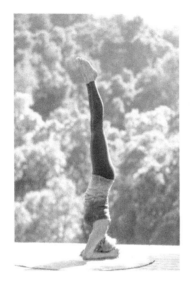

Only practice headstand if it is appropriate for you and you don't have any neck issues or glaucoma. Begin seated, resting your glutes on your heels. Place the elbows on the earth in front of you, shoulder-width apart. Interlace the fingers, and rest the outer edges of the hands on the earth. Gently place the crown of your head on the earth so the head is cradled by your hands. Walk your feet toward your head as far as you can, bending your knees as much as you have to. Slowly send your hips over your shoulders, by drawing, first, one knee to the chest and then the other. Gently untuck the tailbone as you raise your legs to the sky. Feel free to pike up if you can.

In this position, eighty percent of your weight should rest on the arms. That is why it's called a *supported* headstand. It's crucial to find your line upside down in the supported version before moving on to other variations. A lot of the time people dump too much weight onto the cervical or lumbar spine in inversions. It takes practice to be able to position your spine in a way that feels effortless and light when you are upside down. Really engaging your foundation by pushing into the forearms or hands (depending on inversion) and tucking the tailbone ever so slightly will help with this. Your position should feel natural and restful. Please use the wall as long as you need to while practicing headstand.

Benefits: This pose drains the lymphatic system, strengthens the immune system, and tones your core, promoting good posture. Supported headstand directly stimulates the *sahasrara* (crown) *chakra* and helps reverse the direction of the life force in your body. Gravity firmly establishes a downward flow of the life force, towards the earth, in all living beings. Something our physical bodies feel acutely as we age. *Yoga* is concerned with reversing the direction of life force to move up, instead of down. The inversions are one way of achieving that.

RABBIT POSE—SASANGASANA

Start in a tabletop position. Sink your hips to your heels, and place your hands over the outside edges of your feet. Round your spine forward, sending the hips forward and up. Rest the crown of your head gently on the earth as you pull on the outer edges of your feet to deepen the stretch.

Benefits: Rabbit pose provides a shoulder and neck stretch. It stimulates the *sahasrara* (crown *chakra*), your spiritual center and promotes *pratyahara*, withdrawal of the senses.

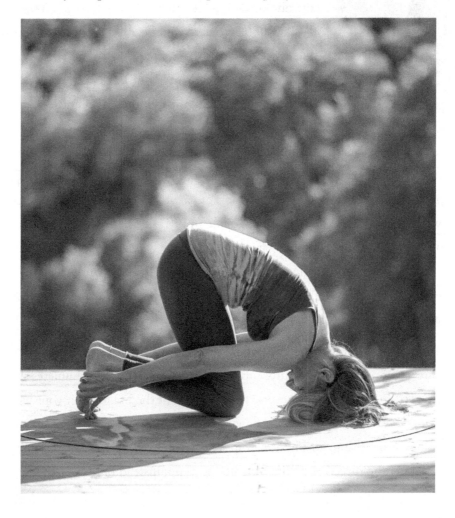

Leila Worby

CORPSE POSE—*SHAVASANA*

For at least five minutes, lie on your back with your arms stretched out by your sides, palms open and facing up. Scan your entire body, slowly moving your attention from your feet to the crown of your head. Notice all the effects of your practice. When you're done, bring your attention to your breath, and sink deeply into your body.

Benefits: The most important pose in *yoga*, corpse pose, provides full-body relaxation and rejuvenation. It allows you to truly reap the benefits of your practice. This is the pose that allows you to cultivate a relationship with your entire subtle body and feel the after effects of your practice. When you start tuning into your subtle body it can feel almost like having a second adolescence. It's best to move into that space with an open mind. You may sense energy in different places that don't exactly correspond to the traditional map of the *chakras*. The commonly used map of the *chakras* draws from many, more elaborated sources.

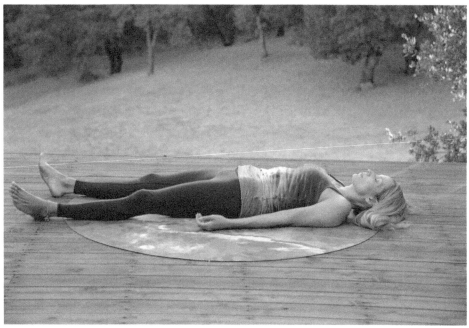

Restorative Poses (Earth)

THREAD THE NEEDLE POSE—*URDHVA MUKHA PASASANA*

Start in a tabletop position. Release your right arm to the side and toward the sky, with your palm facing the earth as you feel the shoulder stretch. Thread your right arm between your left hand and your left knee. To deepen the stretch, release your left arm to the sky, fingertips pointing up.

Benefits: This stretches the shoulder and the neck, and promotes deep relaxation. It stimulates the *anahata* (heart, love, and compassion) *chakra* and the *vishuddhi* (speech and communication) *chakra*.

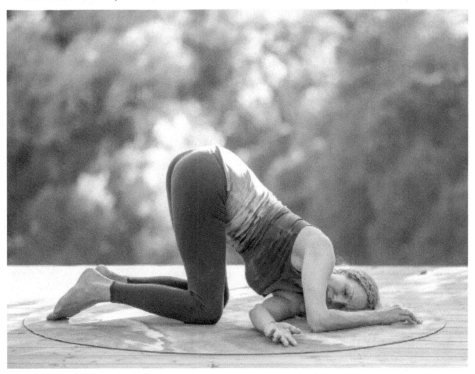

Leila Worby

SUPINE HAND TO TOE POSE—SUPTA HASTA PADANGUSTHASANA

Start in a supine position. Pull your right knee to your chest, and place a strap, if you need to, around the ball of your right foot, or grab the big toe with your peace fingers. Extend the leg up, and pull the foot toward you while gently pressing the sacrum to the earth, finding just the right stretch. You may simultaneously press lightly on your left thigh with your left hand to ground it to the earth.

Benefits: This is a lovely pose to help soothe lower back pain. It stretches the hamstrings and evokes a sense of groundedness and relaxation. Supine hand to toe pose stimulates the *muladhara chakra* (the root and earth center), connecting you with your foundation.

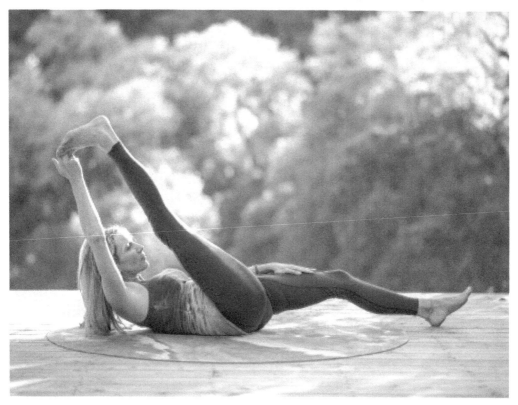

From a supine position on your back, slide your hips to the right slightly, and bring your arms out and away from you. Stretch your right leg over your mid-point and to the left, across your body. You may keep it bent or extend it. Look to the right. You may enjoy the pose here, or if it feels good, you may wrap the right leg around the left, hooking the ankle with the tops of the toes, for *garuda* legs. Take five deep breaths here, letting the scapulae rest flat against the earth.

Benefits: This promotes deep relaxation, aids digestion, and drains the deep lymph nodes and keeps the spine supple. It also restores the spine after deeper backbends. It moves the energy from the *muladhara* (root) to the *sahasrara* (crown) and stimulates the *anahata* (heart) center.

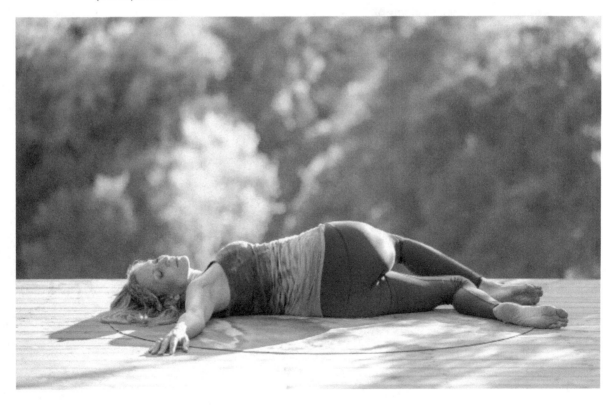

Leila Worby

Sit back with your left leg in front of you and the right leg bent, shin and top of the foot against the earth next to your right hip. Slowly start reclining. Perhaps you are supporting yourself on your palms or on your forearms, or perhaps you can lie all the way back, clasping your elbows. Please listen to your ankles and your knees in this pose, and only go as far as feels good. You may wish to recline on a *yoga* cushion.

Benefits: This pose stretches the quads, hip flexors, and ankles, while promoting relaxation. It stimulates the *svadhisthana chakra* (center of reproductivity and creativity).

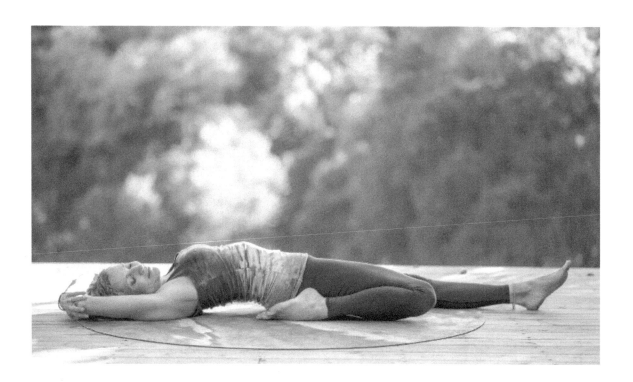

Come to a kneeling position, sit back on the heels of the feet. Widen the knees and place a bolster in front of you as you flow forward. Rest the arms alongside the bolster, and rest the torso, forehead or cheek softly on the bolster. Gaze down and inward.

Benefits: This grounding pose lightly opens the hips, instills profound relaxation, and induces *pratyahara* (withdrawal of the senses). Child's pose stimulates the *muladhara* center, which governs your senses of safety and security. This restorative pose profoundly impacts the nervous system, allowing you to sink even deeper into relaxation.

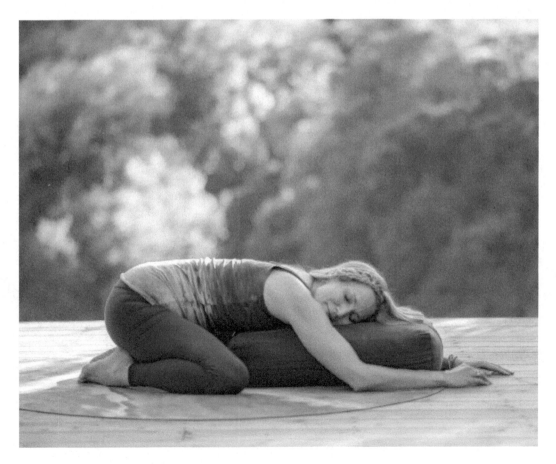

Leila Worby

SUPPORTED FROG POSE—*MANDUKASANA*

Come to a tabletop, facing the long end of your mat. If your knees are sensitive, put a blanket under them. Place a bolster under your lower belly and torso. Slide the knees out so they align with the hips. Keeping your big toes touching. If you want to deepen the stretch, point the toes away from you, with the insides of the feet toward the earth. Ankles aligned with the knees.

Benefits: This pose is a groin and hip opener that stretches the abductors. Frog pose can feel intense for a lot of people, so I love the supported version. When we support our muscles with pillows or props instead of pushing them into uncomfortably deep stretches, they relax and open up naturally. Supported frog pose stimulates the *muladhara* (root) *chakra* and the *svadhisthana* (reproductive) *chakra*.

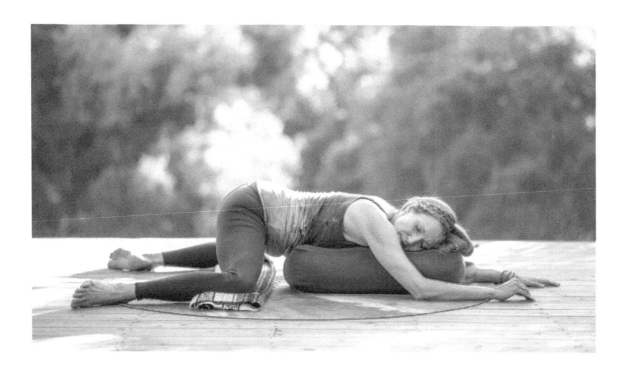

SUPPORTED PIGEON POSE—*SALAMBA KAPOTASANA*

Start in downward-facing dog and draw your right knee to your right wrist. Rest the outer side of the calf onto the earth. Keep your hips parallel, squared to the top of the mat. Rest the outside edge of the foot on the earth, close to the groin. Extend the back leg, with the knee and the top of the foot squared and pressed firmly into the earth. Lift the rib cage to open the heart. Then fold forward and rest the chest on the earth over the forward, bent leg. Support yourself with blankets and a bolster under your hip and forehead as needed.

Benefits: This pose opens the hips and stretches the hip flexors, particularly if you spend a few breaths seated upright, before folding forward. It stimulates the *muladhara* (root) *chakra* and promotes relaxation.

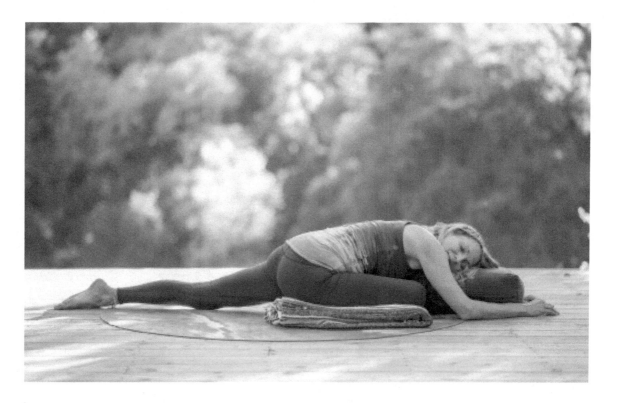

Leila Worby

SUPPORTED BOUND ANGLE POSE—*BADDHA KONASANA*

From a cross legged seated position, bring the soles of the feet together. Bring the heels as close to the groin as possible, keeping the knees close to the ground. Open your feet like a book and fold forward. The shoulders should be pulled back and the spine straight. In this version, we use small pillows or rolled-up blankets to place between the floor and our knees for support, folding forward while resting our torso and forehead, or cheek, on a big bolster.

Benefits: This is a wonderful hip-opening pose that promotes fertility and balances the reproductive system. It supports women during pregnancy and those who may be struggling with hormonal imbalances. Spending more time and really relaxing into this pose in the restorative version, increases the benefits and relaxation. It stimulates the *muladhara* (root) and the *svadhisthana* (reproductive) *chakras.*

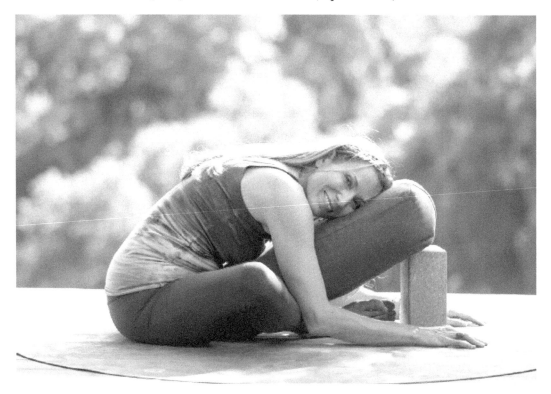

SUPPORTED WIDE-LEGGED FORWARD FOLD— *UPAVISTA KONASANA*

Sit on the earth with your legs stretched out in front of you. Open your legs wide. Place your hands behind you, keeping the fingers pointing away from you, and gently use them to push yourself to the front part of your sitz bones. Fold forward onto a bolster and rest your torso and forehead, or cheek on the bolster.

Benefits: This pose stretches the abductors and the hamstrings. In its full expression it also increases space between the vertebrae of the spine. It stimulates your *svadhisthana chakra*, the center of reproductivity and creativity.

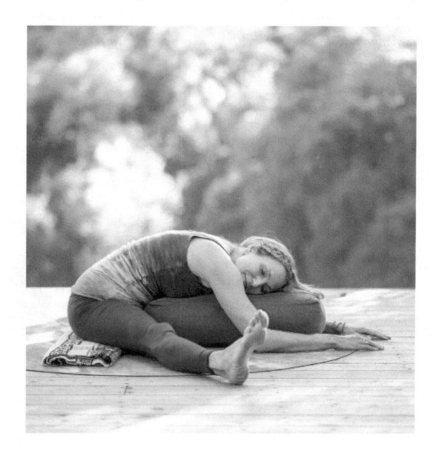

Leila Worby

SUPPORTED FISH POSE—*SALAMBA MATSYASANA*

Start in an easy, seated position (with legs straight out in front of you or bent, with knees falling open to the sides). As you recline, place one block horizontally just underneath your heart, and one block vertically just under your head. If you have an uncomfortable sensation in the lower back, try elevating the sitz bones with a blanket. You can also bring a big bolster to the small of your back and elevate it with blocks at the opposite end and recline on it. Find what works for your body. When this pose feels comfortable you may feel a lovely heart opening and like you can rest in this pose forever.

Benefits: This pose stretches the heart and chest, promoting deep breathing and relaxation. It stimulates the *anahata* (heart) and the *vishuddhi* (throat) *chakras* and aids your connection with your inner essence.

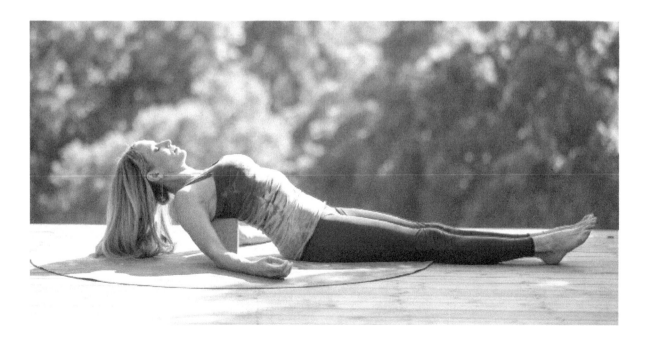

Start in a supine position with your back relaxed on the earth. Extend your legs toward the sky without any tension behind the knees. You may wish to rest them against a wall. Rest the arms alongside the body, and open the palms toward the sky in a receptive mode. Hold this position. The eyes are closed, and the gaze is inward. In some versions, you use the hands to slightly elevate the hips without coming into a full shoulderstand.

Benefits: This pose promotes deep relaxation, aids lymphatic draining, and strengthens the immune system. It stimulates the *ajna* (third eye) *chakra*, the intuitive and psychic center.

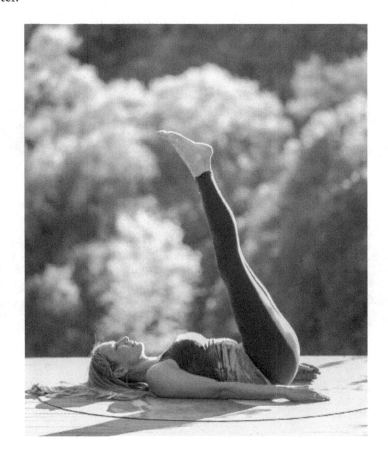

Leila Worby

Standing Poses (For All Elements)

MOUNTAIN POSE—*TADASANA*

This is ground zero, the beginning. When you come into this pose there is an anticipation of action to come. Your senses are alert, and you are preparing to enter flow. To achieve this pose,

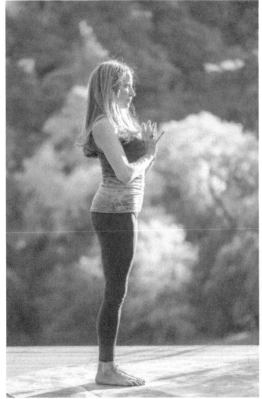

stand straight while maintaining the best posture available to you. Keep your spine straight and the back of your skull aligned with your tailbone. There is an acupressure point in the middle of your soles called "Bubbling Spring." You will know if you're standing with a good posture simply by feeling into this point. If your alignment is correct, it will feel like you popped a bottle of champagne under your feet and as if the bubbles are rising up through the soles of your feet. You need to tuck your tailbone slightly to achieve this sensation.

Benefits: This active standing pose cultivates good posture, strengthens your legs, and grounds you. It further stimulates the *muladhara* (earth) *chakra*.

RAISED HANDS POSE—*URDHVA HASTASANA*

From *tadasana*, reach your arms to the sky and shift your gaze up as well. If it's comfortable for your neck, you may slowly drop your head back. Palms are in a prayer position.

Benefits: This pose slightly stretches your abdominals and, as such, lightly stimulates your digestion. It is a grounding and anticipating pose that stimulates the *muladhara* (earth) center and the *anahata* (heart) center.

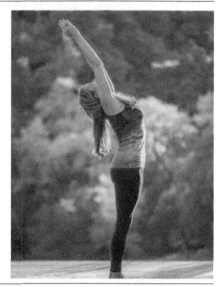

STANDING FORWARD BEND— *UTTANASANA*

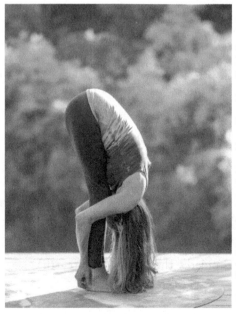

Hinge from the hips and fold forward, attempting to touch your palms to the earth and, eventually, to bring your chest on top of your thighs and your forehead to your shins. You may experiment with grabbing your heels and pulling your torso toward your thighs even more. There is an energetic movement of the skull pulling toward the earth.

Benefits: This pose profoundly stretches the hamstrings. Please be careful here and bend your knees as your hamstring flexibility is developing, so you do not risk injury to your back. Standing forward bend cultivates *pratyahara* (withdrawal of the senses) and deep relaxation. It stimulates the *muladhara* (root) and *svadhisthana* (reproductive) *chakras*.

Leila Worby

STANDING HALF FORWARD BEND—*ARDA UTTANASANA*

From a standing forward fold, come up on the tops of your fingertips and extend your spine straight from your hips. Feel your chest broaden.

Benefits: This stretches the hamstrings and the chest, and it moves grounded energy from the *muladhara* (earth) *chakra* to the *anahata* (heart) *chakra*.

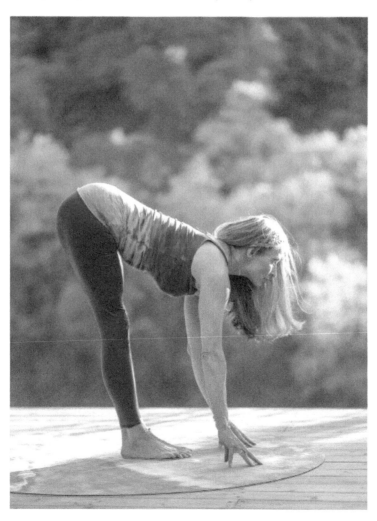

From standing, place the right ankle over the left knee and sit down into your chair pose. Bring your hands into prayer. Breathe here for five slow breaths. .

Benefits: Standing Figure Four opens the hips and promotes balance, strength, and stamina. It stimulates the *muladhara* (root) *chakra* and at the base of the spine, and it relaxes you and makes you feel safe.

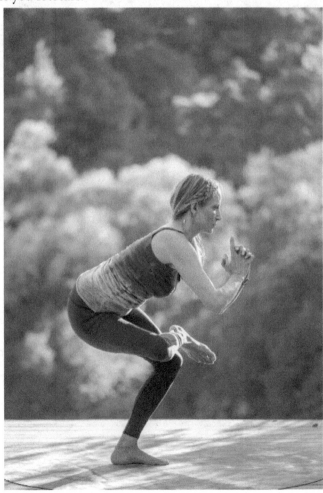

Leila Worby

EAGLE POSE—GARUDASANA

From standing, root down into your right foot. Simultaneously draw your left thigh across your right thigh and your left arm under your right arm. Wrap your limbs and perhaps even hook the foot around the ankle, allowing the palms to meet. Sink into your pose, keeping your spine as erect as possible and your arms and knees aligned toward the center. Squeeze your limbs and explore leaning forward, hinging from the hips and then back to center. Slowly unwrap yourself.

Benefits: This is a lovely shoulder stretch and a balancing pose that stimulates the reproductive system and the libido. It requires open hips and shoulders. The *svadhisthana* (reproductive) and *anahata* (heart) *chakras* are stimulated by spending time in this *asana*.

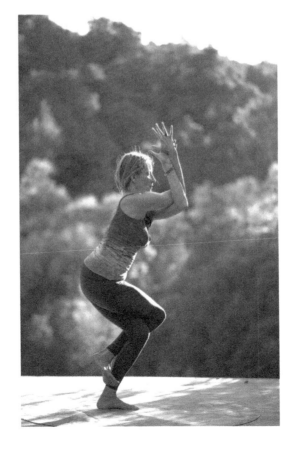

TREE POSE—VRKSASANA

Start from a standing position. Root one foot into the earth. Place the opposite heel on top of the standing foot, or root it into the inner thigh with the toes pointing toward the ground. Tuck the pelvis and the chin. Bring the hands together at the heart in a prayer position. They may also rise over the head. The gaze is forward.

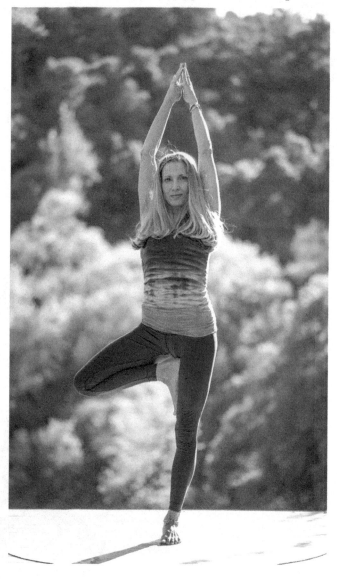

Benefits: Tree Pose promotes balance and focus, and it stretches the hip and the shoulders and increases strength and stamina. It moves the energy from the *muladhara* (root) *chakra* to the *ajna* (third eye) *chakra* and to the *sahasrara* (crown) *chakra*. It allows a movement of energy that starts at the base of your spine (your physical foundation), moves up to your visual and psychic center, and finishes out through your crown. You may think this pose basic, but it's one of the most profound poses of *yoga*.

Leila Worby

STANDING HAND TO TOE VARIATION—*HASTA PADANGUSTASANA*

From tree pose, grab the big toe and extend your leg to the side, then move the leg in front of you. Bow to your leg. Then come back to an upright position with the spine straight, maintaining your leg at a 90-degree angle in front of you. Take three deep breaths here. Slowly lower the foot to the earth.

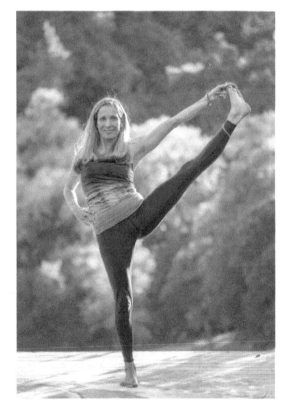

Benefits: This pose promotes balance and focus, and it stretches the hamstrings and the hips. It evokes a sense of groundedness and strength and stimulates the *muladhara chakra* (the root and earth center) and the *ajna* (third eye) *chakra*, promoting clarity of mind and a sense of rootedness.

TRIANGLE POSE—*TRIKONASANA*

From a standing position, step your left foot back into a wide stance, maintaining the legs straight. Point the right toes forward and the back foot at a 45-60 degree angle, toes pointing toward the front. The pelvis is slightly tucked, and the ribcage is lifted.

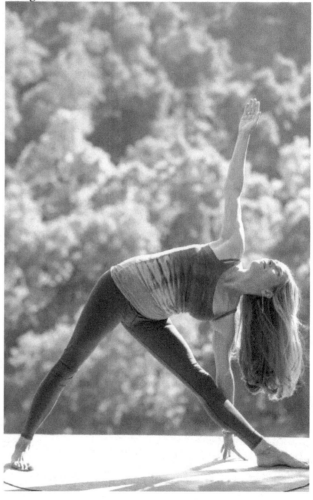

Open sideways, to the right, as you extend your right arm forward and down. Place your hand on the earth, on the outside of your right foot or on your shin. The left arm extends up, toward the sky. Align both arms with the shoulders in a straight line, reaching out with the fingers as the shoulder blades squeeze together. The gaze is toward the top hand. If you have issues with your neck, shift your gaze toward the earth. Press into the outer edge of your back foot.

Benefits: This pose strengthens the legs and stretches the groin, chest, shoulders, and neck. It aids digestion by lightly stretching the abdominals. It stimulates the *muladhara* (root) *chakra*, the *svadhisthana* (reproductive) *chakra* and the *anahata* (heart) *chakra*. Try placing your attention in the heart center when practicing this *asana*.

Leila Worby

EXTENDED SIDE ANGLE—UTTHITA PARSVA KONASANA

From a low lunge with the right foot forward, root the back foot and keep it at a 45-60 degree angle. Open sideways, to the right as you draw your right forearm to your right thigh and spiral the chest open. Stretch the left arm straight overhead and reach forward with the palm facing the earth. You will feel a stretch in your left side waist. If you want to deepen the stretch, place the right hand next to the right foot's outside edge. You can also bind here if you'd like: By bringing the right arm in front of your bent front leg and threading it under the knee, clasping the right wrist with the left hand. Align the crown with the tailbone and the heel.

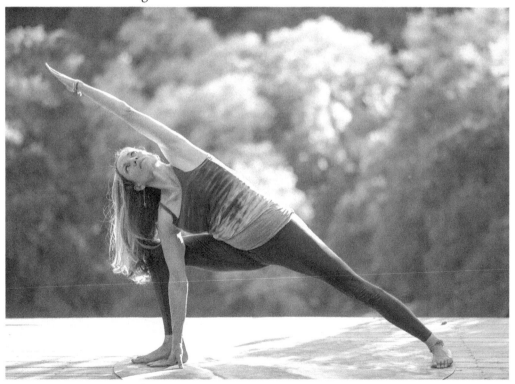

Benefits: This pose builds stamina and strength. It stretches the hips and side waist, and it stimulates the *muladhara* (safety, security, and foundation), *svadhisthana* (creativity and reproduction) and *anahata* (heart, love, and compassion) centers.

Step into a low lunge with your front leg bent in a 90-degree angle, but your knee not traveling over your toes. This is true for all the high lunges. Root your back foot and angle the toes forward at a 45-60-degree angle. The energetic movement here is to press into the outer edge of the back foot and move your hips toward squaring, aligned with the top of the mat. Reach your arms up so they are aligned with your ears. Cup your palms together. If possible, move into a small backbend.

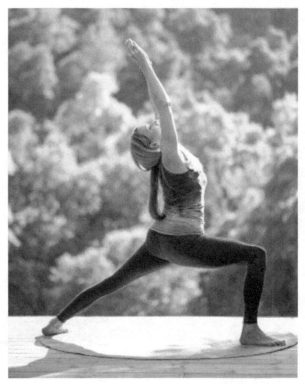

Benefits: This pose stretches the psoas and opens the spine, building strength and stamina. It stimulates the *muladhara* (root), *svadhisthana* (reproductive), and *manipura* (navel and fire) *chakras.*

CRESCENT LOW LUNGE—*ANJANEYASANA*

Low lunge with the back knee dropped. If your lower back is tender, I recommend curling the toes of the back foot under. Place the fingertips on the earth, under your shoulders if that is accessible. Move the sternum forward and up.

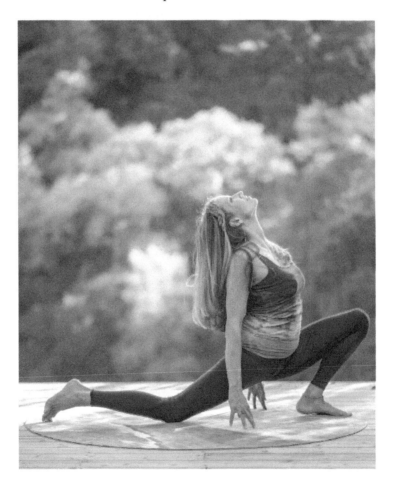

Benefits: This stretches the psoas and the chest and maintains a supple neck and spine. It stimulates the *muladhara* (earth), *svadhisthana* (reproductive), and *anahata* (heart) *chakras.*

CRESCENT LOW LUNGE (CHEST-OPENING)—*ANJANEYASANA*

Low lunge with the back knee dropped. Again-if your lower back is tender, I recommend curling the toes of the back foot under. Raise the arms overhead, against your ears and place your hands in prayer. Move the sternum forward and up.

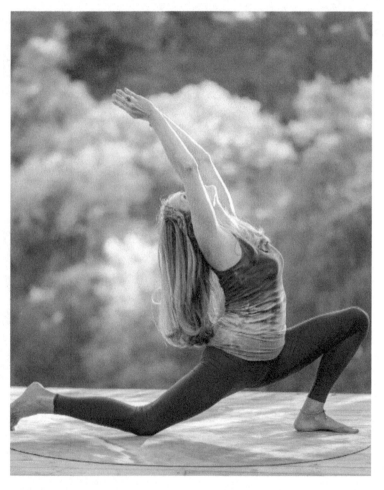

Benefits: This stretches the psoas and the chest and maintains a supple neck and spine. It stimulates the *muladhara* (earth), *svadhisthana* (reproductive), and *anahata* (heart) *chakras*.

Leila Worby

CHAIR POSE—*UTKATASANA*

From standing, bring your feet together, bend your knees, and sit down in an imaginary chair. Lift the toes, and slightly tuck the tailbone. Stretch your arms up and over your head with your hands in prayer.

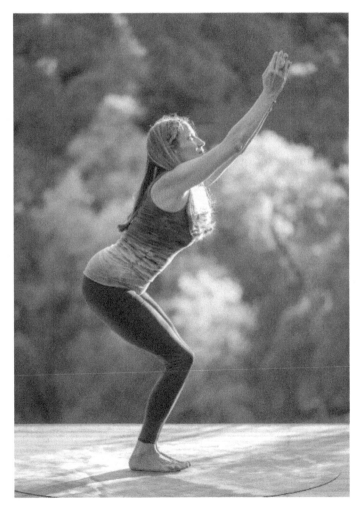

Benefits: This builds strength and stamina, particularly in the glutes. It opens the shoulders and stimulates the *muladhara* (earth) *chakra*.

REVOLVED TRIANGLE POSE—*PARIVRTTA TRIKONASANA*

From a standing position, step the left foot back into a wide stance. Distribute the weight of the body equally between the front and back legs. The legs are parallel and scissor toward each other. The back foot is at a 45-60-degree angle, and the front and back heels are aligned. Reach your left arm up to create space, and then bring the left hand down on the outside of the right foot. Twist your torso and open it toward the sky while squaring the hips as much as possible. Extend the top hand to the sky. If flexibility is limited, place your lower hand on a block positioned against the inner sole of the right foot or your shin. Pull your shoulder blades together and open the arms wide. Gaze toward the thumb in the air or straight ahead if this is not good for your neck.

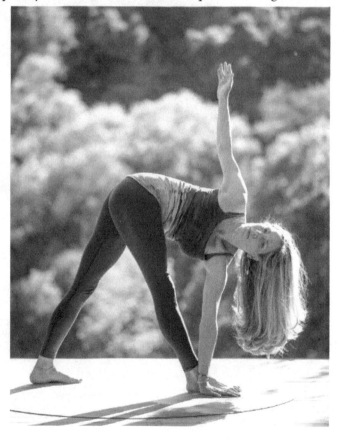

Benefits: This stretches the IT band and hamstrings and builds strength and stamina. It aids digestion, drains the deep lymph nodes, and keeps the spine supple. Revolved triangle pose supports the immune system and prepares the spine for deeper backbends. It also moves the energy from the *muladhara* (root) to the *sahasrara* (crown) and stimulates the *anahata* (heart) center.

Enter this pose from a lunge with your back knee off the earth. Traditionally, the back foot is rooted, but it's easier to come up on the ball of the back foot. Start with the right foot forward and reach your left hand to the sky. Exhale and start by hooking the left elbow over the right thigh, bringing your hands into prayer. Maybe even place the left hand on the outside of the right foot, or on a block placed outside the foot. You can open your arms wide, or you may wish to bind here for a deeper shoulder stretch: thread your left arm under your right thigh, wrapping your right arm around your own waist and clasping the fingertips of the left hand with the fingertips of your right hand or even the wrist.

Benefits: This pose builds strength and stamina, and stretches the hip flexors. It aids digestion, drains the deep lymph nodes, and keeps the spine supple, preparing the body for deeper backbends. It moves the energy from the *muladhara* (root) to the *sahasrara* (crown) and stimulates the *anahata* (heart) center.

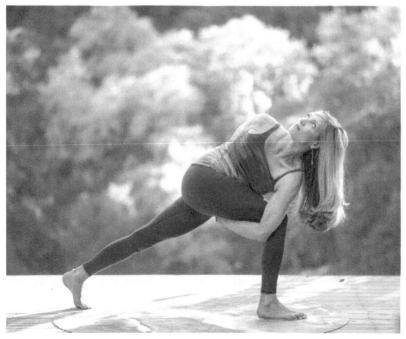

REVOLVED CHAIR POSE—*PARSVA UTKATASANA*

Inhale as you sweep your hands up. Bend your knees and sit down into an imaginary chair. Tuck your tailbone slightly as you draw your belly button to your spine, and lift the toes from the earth. On an exhale, twist the torso to the right, keeping the knees in one line. Place your left elbow against the outer side of the right knee. Form a fist with your left hand and press your right palm into it and extend your right arm to the sky. Gaze to the sky. Maybe extend your arms to the sides, like wings. Inhale back to chair pose and exhale.

Benefits: This pose aids digestion, drains the deep lymph nodes, supports the immune system, and keeps the spine and neck supple. It strengthens the glutes and hamstrings and prepares the spine for deeper backbends. Revolved chair pose moves the energy from the *muladhara* (root) to the *sahasrara* (crown) and stimulates the *anahata* (heart) center.

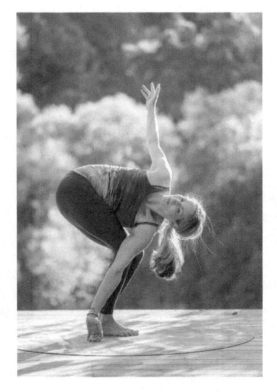

Leila Worby

CHAPTER 6

Curated Practices

This section contains customized practices that outline the most impactful options of all the techniques (*pranayama*, *mantra*, *mudra*, *meditation*, *namaskar and asana*) described in this book, to bring your unique body back to balance.

Sarva Mangalam! Auspiciousness on your new beginning!

SATTVA-ENHANCING PRACTICE

These practices are for you if you feel balanced and happy most of the time, but you just want to enhance your already healthy life with a personal *yoga* practice, beyond the poses of yoga. If you are someone who has taken a lot of classes in the past, but are ready to explore a full yoga practice that's entirely your own, this is a good place to start.

When I first discovered the poses of *yoga*, I did them out of a book for years. There were no fancy *Yoga* Studios in Europe at the time. What's nice about using a book as your guide, is that you don't end up going too deep into poses, trying to subconsciously imitate the teacher's expression of the pose, because you can't take your time to fully explore it. It additionally teaches you to move on your own breath and at your own phase, without having to keep up with a group. You can play around, take as many breaks as you feel like. Wear whatever feels comfortable and look as silly as you want in the privacy and comfort of your own living room. That is a much more conducive environment to turning your attention inwards. When you practice with other people their practice and energy can at times be distracting and guide your attention outside of yourself. It's easier to be driven by the ego in that environment instead of relaxing into your inner essence.

- Five-Minute *Pranayama* Practice—*Nadi Shodhana*

- Five-Minute *Mudra* Practice—*Svabhava Mudra*

- Fifteen-Minute *Namaskar* Practice—Classical *Namaskar*

- Fifteen-Minute Postural Practice

Locust Pose—*Shalabhasana*

Bow Pose (Optional)—*Dhanurasana*

Triangle Pose—*Trikonasana*

Revolved Triangle Pose—*Parivrtta Trikonasana*

Tree Pose—*Vrksasana*

Boat Pose—*Navasana*

Hero's Pose—*Virasana*

Bridge Pose—*Sethu Bandha Sarvangasana*

Reverse Table Pose—*Ardha Purvottanasana OR*

Upward Bow Pose (Optional)—*Urdhva Dhanurasana*

Rabbit Pose—*Sasangasana OR*

Supported Headstand (Optional)—*Salamba Sirsasana*

Feet up the Wall—*Viparita Karani OR*

Shoulderstand (Optional)—*Salamba Sarvangasana*

Corpse Pose—*Shavasana*

- Five-Minute Goddess Meditation

RAJAS-PACIFYING PRACTICE

When you are ruled by *rajas*, the temptation is to go running or to complete a strong *yoga* practice. However, in this situation, what your body needs is to slow down and relax. As mentioned before, if you are suffering from excess *rajas*, which expresses itself as racing, shattered thoughts, excessive worry, anxiety, and panic attacks. Choose from the following *pranayamas*, *namaskars*, and poses. You don't want to stimulate *rajas* even further. You want to encourage your Parasympathetic Nervous System as much as you can to achieve balance, and you want to use the force of gravity to surrender into a more grounded and harmonious state.

In addition to practicing *pranayama* to calm the mind, before going to bed, take a nice bath or shower to calm down, and turn off your screen an hour and a half before bedtime. You may also wish to start writing a short to-do list for the coming day. Get all your worrying thoughts on paper. This way, all the thoughts circulating in your mind are on paper. They are safe there. You can let go of them now as you close the book and climb under the covers.

- Viloma pranayama

- Bhramari Pranayama, or "Bumblebee Breath" (for insomnia)

Reminder: *Bhramari pranayama* should not be practiced by pregnant or menstruating women. It is also contraindicated for high blood pressure, epilepsy, chest pain, or an active ear infection.

- Five-Minute *Apan Vayu Mudra* Practice

- Fifteen-Minute *Chandra Namaskar*

- Fifteen-Minute Postural Practice

Child's Pose—*Balasana*

Cat/Cow Pose—*Marjaryasana/Bitilasana*

Seated Forward Fold *Paschimottanasana*

One Leg Folded Forward Bend—*Trianga Mukaikapada Paschimottanasana*

Head to Knee Pose—*Janu Sirsasana*

Seated Twist—*Parivrtta Sukhasana*

Bound Angle Pose—*Baddha Konasana*

Wide-Legged Forward Fold—*Upavistha Konasana*

Tortoise Pose—*Kurmasana*

Bridge Pose—*Sethu Bandha Sarvangasana*

Feet Up the Wall—*Viparita Karani OR*

Shoulderstand (Optional)—*Salamba Sarvangasana*

Plow Pose (Optional)—*Halasana*

Supine Twist—*Supta Matsyendrasana*

Supported Fish Pose—*Salamba Matsyasana*

Corpse Pose—*Shavasana*

- Five-Minute Goddess Meditation

TAMAS-PACIFYING PRACTICE

If you are suffering from a *tamas* imbalance, you are in a deep state of inertia. You feel dull, slow, and heavy. You might be experiencing a deep state of depression. If your depression feels more rooted in anxiety versus the monotonous, weightiness that characterize *tamas*, I would recommend the *Rajas*-pacifying practice outlined above instead.

Again, please see these suggestions as complementary to any treatment you are currently undergoing. Always consult a doctor before undertaking any of the practices in this book, and listen to your body to see how the practices affect you.

Sometimes when we are down, it's hard to even get out of bed, let alone do a rigorous *yoga* practice. But if you're not yet too deep in the grips of *tamas*, a *yoga* practice will energize you and bring you back to life. Even if you only do five minutes of *pranayama*, you will be taking an important step forward. If the *namaskar is* too strong for you, do the *chandra namaskar* or the classical *namaskar* with the *bija mantras* outlined in Chapter 3. But if you can summon the strength to do a full *surya namaskar*, it will snap you out of *tamas* quickly. Before commencing the *pranayama* I recommend a few minutes of awareness practice. This will allow your breathing to deepen organically.

- Five-Minute Full-Body Relaxation

- Five-Minute Bhastrika Pranayama

Reminder: If you suffer from any heart problems or elevated blood pressure, or are pregnant or menstruating, please do not undertake this *pranayama* but do *surya bhedana pranayama* instead.

Leila Worby

- Surya Bhedana Pranayama

- Omkar Kriya with Mantra

- Five-Minute Prana Mudra Practice OR

- Surya Mudra Practice

- Fifteen-Minute Surya Namaskar

I recommend three rounds of *surya namaskar* A, and three to five rounds of *surya namaskar* B.

- Fifteen-Minute Postural Practice

Child's Pose—*Balasana*

Cat/Cow Pose—*Marjaryasana/Bitilasana*

Balancing Table—*Uttitha Marjaryasana*

Thread the Needle Pose—*Urdhva Mukha Pasasana*

Knees-Chest-Chin Pose—*Ashtanga Namaskara*

Locust Pose—*Shalabhasana*

Bow Pose—*Dhanurasana*

Half Lord of the Fishes—*Ardha Matsyendrasana*

Hero's Pose—*Virasana*

Camel Pose—*Ustrasana*

Boat Pose—*Navasana*

Yogic Squat—*Malasana*

Crow Pose (Optional)—*Bakasana*

Bridge Pose—*Sethu Bandha Sarvangasana*

Upward Bow Pose (Optional)—*Urdhva Dhanurasana*

Rabbit Pose—*Sasangasana OR*

Supported Headstand (Optional)—*Salamba Sirsasana*

ShoulderStand (Optional)—*Salamba Sarvangasana*

Plow Pose (Optional)—*Halasana*

Corpse Pose—*Shavasana*

- Five-Minute Goddess Meditation

PRACTICES FOR INCREASED FOCUS AND ATTENTION

If you have ever had a hard time concentrating or absorbing mundane information, these practices are for you. Always remember to take a few deep breaths, focusing your attention exclusively on the breath at any point during your day when you feel your attention shattering. Those of us with a sensitive constitution easily feel overwhelmed with sensory information, which may lead to an agitated state, preventing us from processing information. It's like the brain is experiencing scratches in its grooves (if I were to liken the brain to an old vinyl record), which makes it hard to overcome thoughts and move on. This makes it almost impossible to structure our thoughts and speech. To combat this state, calming the nervous system is key as is practicing *dharana* (focus) meditations.

Leila Worby

- SOHAM Kriya (focus)

- Trataka on Candle

- Five-Minute Hakini Mudra Practice

- Surya namaskars A and B

- Fifteen-Minute Postural Practice

Child's Pose—*Balasana*

Cat/Cow Pose—*Marjaryasana/Bitilasana*

Balancing Table—*Uttitha Marjaryasana*

Side Plank—*Vasisthasana*

Knees-Chest-Chin Pose—*Ashtanga Namaskara*

Locust Pose—*Shalabhasana*

Half Frog Pose—*Arda Bhekasana*

Bow Pose—*Dhanurasana*

Half Lord of the Fishes—*Ardha Matsyendrasana*

Boat Pose—*Navasana*

Yogic Squat—*Malasana*

Crow Pose (Optional)—*Bakasana*

Revolved Chair -Pose—*Parsva Utkatasana*

Side Crow Pose (Optional)—*Parsva Bakasana*

Handstand Jumps (Optional)—*Adho Mukha Vrksasana*

Bridge Pose—*Sethu Bandha Sarvangasana*

Upward Bow Pose (Optional)—*Urdhva Dhanurasana*

Rabbit Pose—*Sasangasana OR*

Supported Headstand—*Salamba Sirsasana*

Shoulderstand (Optional)—*Salamba Sarvangasana*

Plow Pose (Optional)—*Halasana*

Corpse Pose—*Shavasana*

- Five-Minute Goddess Meditation

PRACTICE FOR OVERCOMING ADDICTION AND SUPPORTING SELF ACCEPTANCE

These practices are for anyone who struggles with addiction to food, alcohol, drugs, gambling, sex, or harmful relationships. Addiction stems from a misguided effort to fill the inner void and digest overwhelming emotions.

The goal of this practice is to trigger the Parasympathetic Nervous System, which will slow you down and help you control your impulses. The square breathing *pranayama* will additionally train the brain to take one step at a time, something that can seem impossible when in the deep grip of addiction. The *mudras* and poses recommended here will help you cultivate self-love and self-confidence and aid you in digesting strong emotions. The entire practice will help you connect with the life force, the missing piece of the puzzle that you have been looking for outside of yourself. Overcoming addiction is like walking through fire. If you are struggling with addiction, I highly recommend that you seek out a support group and a strong mentor. You must lean on others until the fire has died down a bit and you're strong enough to walk alone. I am holding you in my prayers.

- Square Breathing—*Pranayama*

- Five-Minute *Vajrapadma Mudra* Practice

- Five-Minute *Bhumisparsa Mudra* Practice

Please note that this is a variation of the traditional *bhumisparsa mudra*, and it is aimed at soothing the emotional body, unlike the traditional, which is used for spiritual awakening.

- Fifteen-Minute *Chandra Namaskar*

- Fifteen-Minute Postural Practice

Cat/Cow Pose—Marjaryasana/Bitilasana

Thread the Needle Pose—Urdhva Mukha Pasasana

Reclined Half Hero's Pose—Supta Ardha Virasana

Bow Pose—Dhanurasana

Camel Pose—Ustrasana

Seated Forward Fold—Paschimottanasana

Head to Knee Pose—Janu Sirsasana

Supported Bound Angle Pose—Baddha Konasana

Supported Wide-Legged Forward Fold—Upavista Konasana

Feet up the Wall—Viparita Karani

Shoulderstand (Optional)—Salamba Sarvangasana

Supported Fish Pose—Salamba Matsyasana

Corpse -Pose—Shavasana

- Five Minute Goddess Meditation

PRACTICES TO INCREASE FERTILITY

These practices are intended to support the female reproductive system and hormones at any age. As a prenatal *yoga* teacher, I have customized *yoga* practices for women trying to conceive and balance their hormonal bodies before and after the child bearing years. I have indicated which poses should not be practiced during pregnancy. .

Yogic practices should complement an existing fertility treatment to increase the enjoyment of this special time in your life. If you're struggling with fertility, please know you are perfect just the way you are. You do not have to become or perform to fulfill your purpose on this earth. You are enough just as you are. Please try not to lose sight of your experience of being alive through all of this.

CALLING ON THE SPIRIT OF YOUR CHILDREN

The moment I knew I was ready to get pregnant, I called on the souls of my children. A creature who thrives on habits, I walked along a beautiful trail in the Northern California Bay Area every evening. Walking can put you in a deep state of flow because of the repetitive movement it requires. Every evening, I spoke to the soul of my future child, saying I was ready and excited to meet him or her and for all the little things we would do together. I told this soul of my future I was warm and cozy and that it was time for us to meet each other. I was lucky enough to fall pregnant very quickly with each of my sons.

When my oldest son was about three years old, I took him for a walk down the same trail. We had moved away from the area, so it was the first time he'd come down that trail. He looked at me and said, "Mommy, I remember seeing you and your big belly from above. I was hovering in the treetops, and I decided to jump into your belly to wake you up." And he sure has kept me awake and on my toes ever since.

Calling on the spirit of your child might sound silly or meaningless, but I do believe it prepares your mind and your physical being for pregnancy. I also think our children's spirits can hear us calling to them. To do this, you don't need a ritual. You just need to do it whenever you feel yourself in a creative flow or when you feel relaxed in nature.

- Pranayamas

I recommend a five-minute *pranayama: nadi shodhana*, *viloma*, or square breathing. Bring one, or maybe even all three, into your daily routine. Clary sage essential oil is known to balance estrogen, so it may boost fertility. You may also wish to use sandalwood and lavender if you feel like your stress levels need to come down.

- Five-Minute *Mudra* Practices

Shakti Mudra

Yoni Mudra

Chandra Namaskar (Change transition from ashtanga pranam and cobra to chaturanga dandasana and upward-facing dog as long as you feel strong enough when pregnant.)

- **Fifteen-Minute Postural Practice**

Standing Figure Four—*Eka Pada Utkatasana*

Eagle Pose—*Garudasana* (not advised during pregnancy)

Yogic Squat—*Malasana*

Cobra Pose—*Bhujangasana* (not advised during pregnancy)

Bow Pose—*Dhanurasana* (not advised during pregnancy)

Supported Bound Angle Pose—*Baddha Konasana*

Supported Wide-Legged Forward Fold—*Upavista Konasana*

Supported Frog Pose—*Mandukasana*

Bridge Pose—*Sethu Bandha Sarvangasana* (not advised during pregnancy)

Supported Fish Pose—*Salamba Matsyasana*

Shoulderstand (Optional)—*Salamba Sarvangasana* (not advised during pregnancy)

Plow Pose (Optional)—*Halasana* (not advised during pregnancy)

Supine Twist—*Supta Matsyendrasana* (not advised during pregnancy)

Corpse Pose—*Shavasana* (when pregnant, you can lie on your left side)

- **Five-Minute Goddess Meditation**

Leila Worby

PRACTICES FOR THE MOON AND SOLAR JUNCTIONS

It's useful to surf the energies of the sun and the moon cycles and use them to your advantage. Doing so will strengthen your subtle body and make you more attuned to it at the same time. Do these practices to take advantage of the heightened energies at the times of the solstices, equinoxes, and full and new moons. These junctions are considered particularly auspicious for *sadhana* or spiritual practice. You can use the new moon practice at the time of the winter solstice and the full moon practice at the time of the summer solstice if they resonate with you.

NEW MOON PRACTICE

The new moon, represented by the bottom of an exhale, is a time for a fresh start. It is also a time when there is very little lunar energy, so it's common to feel the strong pull of the earth's energies at this time, often through a heavy, slow, lethargic feeling. When the moon is new, it's a perfect time to slow down, turn inward, and listen to your needs and what you want to bring forth for the next cycle. We can learn to listen deeply by learning to slow down and surrender fully. During this time, long holds in poses in which your body is supported by the earth are usually the best option. Full-body surrender, restorative, and *Yin* practices are perfect during the new moon. You will find concrete suggestions under the curated practice below.

There are some really lovely *mantras* to listen to and flow to during the time of the new moon. One of my personal favorites is the *Adi Shakti mantra*.

I always like to start a new moon practice by smudging myself with sage to clear my body. This ritual can be used any time, especially when you feel drowned by the negative energies of toxic events, people, or places. Smudging is like an energy shower. The best *namaskar* for the new moon is *chandra namaskar*. Practice this at night with lit candles. After about fifteen to twenty minutes of enjoying this *namaskar*, do some or all of the poses listed below.

To conclude your new moon practice, take as long as you need to journal about your intentions for the next cycle. If your wildest dreams could come true, what would they look like? What concrete steps can you take to achieve these goals? How can these steps be broken down into daily and weekly goals? Take a few moments to visualize a reality in which your plans have come true. It's good to do this visualization every evening just before you go to sleep.

- Adi Shakti Mantra

- Chandra Namaskar

- Poses for the New Moon

Restorative Child's Pose—*Balasana*

Supported Pigeon Pose—*Salamba Kapotasana*

Supported Bound Angle Pose—*Baddha Konasana*

Supported Wide-Legged Forward Fold—*Upavista Konasana*

Supported Frog Pose—*Mandukasana*

Supine Hand to Toe—*Supta Hasta Padangusthasana*

Supine Twist—*Supta Matsyendrasana*

Supported Fish Pose—*Salamba Matsyasana**

Corpse Pose—*Shavasana* (for at least five minutes)

- Five-Minute Goddess Meditation

* If you can only do one pose, do this one.

Leila Worby

FULL MOON PRACTICE

The full moon is represented by the top of the inhale. Now is a time for gratitude, fullness, and letting go. It is common to feel very energized and ungrounded during this time as the lunar energies draw you toward the moon. Most people have a hard time sleeping through the night and are kept up by the moon's gorgeous fullness and luminescence. At this time, I absolutely love to do longer, more robust practices. I usually start with three *surya namaskar* As and then do as many sun salutation Bs as I want. When my strength buckles, I move into standing poses, grounding forward folds, and hip openers.

After your long *shavasana*, grab your journal and write down everything for which you are grateful in your life. Evaluate what has come to a culmination in your life, particularly during this moon cycle. It might be useful to refer back to your journaling on the new moon. What adjustments do you need to make to achieve your goals? What elements in your life cause discord? What stressors would you like to let go of? Once you have written your list, roll up the page and burn it, either in your fireplace or over the sink. Then, take a long, rejuvenating Epsom salts bath, scented with lavender, before you enjoy your moon bath.

MOON BATHING

An ancient *yogic* practice I have come to love is Moon Bathing. You wrap yourself up warmly, go outside, and sit or lie under the full moon for thirty minutes to an hour. Bathing in her energy. I like to do a few moments of *SOHAM kriya*, with the moon as the focal point. You can also practice gazing at the full moon, which is said to be incredibly powerful for fine-tuning your hormone system. It's similar to trataka on a candle, but with the moon as your focal point. However, you don't have to do anything but breathe, letting your endocrine and nervous systems balance themselves by soaking up the lunar light and energy. Visualize the full moon filling you up with *amrita* or divine lunar nectar. If you have a lot of energy during a full moon, you may choose to take a long walk. The full moon creates a time of intense energy, so I like to do a strong practice with many grounding poses, such as hip openers and forward folds. You will find suggested poses below.

- *Purnamadah Mantra* for the Full Moon

- *Surya Namaskars* A and B

- Poses for the Full Moon

Standing Figure Four—*Eka Pada Utkatasana*

Tree Pose—*Vrksasana*

Standing Hand to Toe Variation—*Hasta Padangustasana*

Triangle Pose—*Trikonasana*

Revolved Triangle Pose—*Parivrtta Trikonasana*

Extended Side Angle—*Utthita Parsva Konasana*

Revolved Side Angle—*Parivrtta Parsvakonasana*

Wide-Legged Forward Fold—*Prasarita Padottanasana*

Yogic Squat—*Malasana*

Firefly Pose—*Tittibasana*

Locust Pose—*Shalabhasana*

Half Frog Pose—*Arda Bhekasana*

Bow Pose—*Dhanurasana*

Camel Pose—*Ustrasana*

Bridge Pose—*Sethu Bandha Sarvangasana*

Upward Bow Pose (Optional)—*Urdhva Dhanurasana*

Supine Twist—*Supta Matsyendrasana*

Seated Forward Fold—*Paschimottanasana*

Head to Knee Pose—*Janu Sirsasana*

Seated Twist—*Bharadvajasana*

Rabbit Pose—*Sasangasana OR*

Supported Headstand—*Salamba Sirsasana*

Feet up the Wall—*Viparita Karani OR*

Shoulderstand (Optional)—*Salamba Sarvangasana*

Corpse Pose—*Shavasana*

- Five-Minute Goddess Meditation

CRAFTING A *YOGIC* PRACTICE THAT FITS YOUR LIFESTYLE

When we live disconnected from life force, we are constantly out of sync with nature, and our lives feel boring and without purpose. Suppose we have developed an imbalanced nervous system. In that case, we can, as outlined earlier, be troubled by anxiety, panic attacks, and deep states of burnout and depression. When we are imbalanced, we may struggle with elementary tasks, such as getting out of bed in the morning.

Completing a *yoga* practice can seem daunting, maybe even impossible. The good news is that you still have your breath, and you can always do five minutes a day of breathing exercises that will literally *breathe* the life force back into you. And once you have more life force, you can add additional practices to further your well-being.

It only takes five minutes to start a new habit. You will tailor your practice according to your schedule and the techniques that have the most profound effect on you. In my experience, the best thing to do is to really immerse yourself in *yoga* during a retreat for five days or so, time and resource-permitting. Retreats allow you to immerse yourself immediately and connect with the life force. Once you establish a connection with life force, it is easy to drop into it and maintain it in your life with shorter practices. Below are several examples of practices with suggested times, listed in order of difficulty from the least challenging to the most challenging. For each practice, choose the *pranayamas*, *mudras*, *namaskars*, and poses that work for you. In the beginning, I recommend doing at least twenty minutes of practice every day.

PRACTICE 1 (10-MINUTE EXPRESS PRACTICE— BECAUSE A LITTLE BIT IS BETTER THAN NOTHING)

- 5-minute *pranayama*

- 5-minute *mudra* practice

PRACTICE 2 (20-MINUTE PRACTICE— IF YOU FIND PHYSICAL ACTIVITY CHALLENGING)

- 10-minute *pranayama*
- 5-minute *mudra* practice

- 5-minute Goddess Meditation

PRACTICE 3 *(20-MINUTE PRACTICE— IF YOU WISH TO INCORPORATE MOVEMENT)

- 5-minute pranayama

- 15-minute namaskar practice

PRACTICE 4 (60-MINUTE PRACTICE)*

- 5-15-minute *pranayama*

- 5-15-minute *mudra* practice

- 30-50-minute *namaskar* and postural practice

- 5-10-minute Goddess Meditation

- 5-10-minute *shavasana*

* If you wish to create a more physically challenging practice, please do *namaskars* before the poses. They will warm up your body and prepare it to safely enter the poses. And as always, please consult with your doctor before embarking on any of the practices described in this book.

Leila's Recommendations

EASY *KITCHARI* RECIPE

Ingredients

1 tablespoon coconut oil or ghee
2 teaspoons mustard seeds
1 teaspoon cumin seeds
1 yellow onion, diced (yields about 1 1/3 cups)
3 carrots, peeled and diced
1 tablespoon minced ginger
2 cloves garlic, minced
1 teaspoon salt
1 teaspoon ground turmeric
1/4 teaspoon ground cloves
1/4 teaspoon ground black pepper
3/4 cup basmati or jasmine rice, rinsed
1 cup dried moong dal or red lentils, rinsed
4 cups vegetable broth
2 cups water

Instructions

1) Heat the coconut oil or ghee in a heavy-bottomed pot over medium heat. Add the mustard seeds and cumin seeds and toast them until the mustard seeds start to pop (about 1 to 2 minutes). Add the onions, carrots, ginger, and garlic. Cook for about 5 minutes, stirring frequently to keep the vegetables and spices from burning.

2) Once the onions have softened, add the salt, turmeric, cloves, and black pepper and stir until the spices coat the vegetables. Add the rice, moong dal, vegetable broth, and water. Bring everything to a boil, then reduce the heat to low. Cover the pot and simmer the *kitchari* for about 20 minutes. After 15 minutes of

cooking, check to see if there is still enough liquid in the pot. If you notice that the liquid is completely absorbed by the rice and beans, add 1/2 to 1 cup of water and stir to incorporate.

3) Remove the lid and check to see if the rice is tender. If the *kitchari* looks too runny, let it simmer, uncovered, for a few more minutes. If the *kitchari* is too thick, turn off the heat, add 1/2 to 1 cup of water, and stir. Taste and see if you need to add a small pinch of salt.

4) Serve the *kitchari* in bowls, along with chili oil, cilantro, and lemon wedges, if you like.

Nutrition Information

Serves 4, amount per serving: Calories: 398, Total Fat 5.4g, Saturated Fat: 3.2g, Cholesterol: 0mg, Sodium: 1174mg, Total Carbohydrate: 73.3g, Dietary Fiber: 8.5g, Sugar: 6.7g, Protein 15.6g

MANTRAS

One of the most well-known, classic recordings of the *Gayatri mantra* is Deva Premal and Mitten's. I recommend searching it up and listening to it during your practice.

You will find many versions of the *Adi Shakti mantra*. I recommend Nirinjan Kau's version. But pick your own.

Shantala has a beautiful recording of *Purnamadah* that I recommend listening to during your full moon practice.

CONCLUSION

The techniques in this book are drawn from many ancient *yogic* scriptures I have come to rely on in my studies and practice. Some of my favorites include *The Yoga Sutras*, *Gheranda Samhita*, *Shiva Samhita*, *Hatha Yoga Pradipika*, *The Vijnana Bhairava Tantra*, and *The Recognition Sutras*. They have been tested in my own personal practice. I've seen them benefit my students, too. In my own practice, I use all of these techniques, depending on how much energy I have available and what my being needs at any particular moment.

Once you have established a practice using this book's options and recommendations, feel free to branch out and try them all. Never limit yourself to just one style of practice. You will learn over time when to use what type of practice by listening inward to what your physical and subtle bodies require. The important thing is that you look forward to your practice. It should be your haven and your sanctuary, your place of refuge. Suppose you are suffering from emotional discord during your day. Five minutes can work miracles to shift your emotional state, especially if you use a technique grounded in an established everyday practice. *Yoga* is a movement from the gross to the subtle. The human experience is changing from moment to moment, and your experience is always unfolding just as it should. Do your best to move into that quiet space within yourself where real magic happens through these practices. I hope the techniques in this book will serve you on your path. I am honored to have been able to share them with you.

HOW YOGA BECAME MY PATH

I grew up on the icy, rainy shores of western Sweden, in Kattegat, a region known for Viking raids that occurred over a thousand years ago. Growing up, I listened as my grandmother told tales of all the great Aesir gods. I was fascinated by religion and spirituality. I had read most of the esoteric and primary scriptures of the main world religions by the time I was out of high

Leila Worby

school. The main world religions commonly refers to Buddhism, Christianity, Islam, Hinduism and Judism.

My grandmother's stories taught me at an early age how the various gods and goddesses in the Aesir mythology represented different energies and qualities important to the formation of the human psyche as well as the powers that are essential to survival and understanding one's surroundings. This integrated knowledge made understanding the deep origins and significance of the *Tantric* gods and goddesses natural and intuitive when I began to study *Yoga* and *Tantra* in depth. It was as though my early life had prepared me for the path that lay ahead.

I was a big hippie during my teenage years. My nickname was "Barefoot Leila," which made sense—I walked around barefoot most of the time. In my mind, John Lennon was the closest thing to the next Messiah. It was as though I was subconsciously drawn to the art of the Beatles because of its undercurrent of Easter spirituality and non-duality.

I thought, if I could only find their Guru in India or study at one of the ashrams in Rishikesh, I would be able to leave behind the gross experience of life and transcend to a place of lightness and joy that I intuitively knew existed but had no clue how to reach. I was thinking of *utkranti*—the final act of an enlightened *yogi* leaving his body—long before I heard the word.

After high school, during a three-months' backpacking trip in India, I had profound experiences of oneness with the universe. I lived in complete flow, and I felt guided by a higher force. I subsisted on fresh fruit on the beaches of Gujarat and looked forward to finding an ashram where I could learn more about meditation. At this time I was not interested at all in the poses, although I had experienced them.

Unfortunately, my trip to India was cut short. I fell off a cliff and broke my spine in seventy places, mainly the lower part of my spine, the tailbone, and the pubic bones—the actual seat of the life force in *yogic* philosophy. I also broke my right arm and was airlifted home without knowing if I would ever move my legs again. The irony of the accident was that I had gone to India in search of transcendence but was firmly pulled back into the reality of my very mortal and very fleeting embodied experience.

Years passed, and I completed my master's degree in Social Science. I took a position working for Google in a fast-paced environment. It wasn't until I became pregnant with my first son in 2010, that I fell deep into *yoga*. I had taken my first *yoga* class at age sixteen and practiced regularly for years before that, but I did not have a personal, everyday home practice. During my pregnancy, *yoga* finally clicked for me. It slowed me down and relaxed me. It grounded me deep into my body and allowed me to drop-in and fully inhabit it. Until then, I had always felt like I was walking outside of my body, observing myself from the outside. This is an experience that is often triggered by stress. For me, this alienation from self was a result of a fast-paced lifestyle and the trauma to my body years earlier.

After experiencing *yoga's* transformative power, I started studying it in more detail. I became a regular at Esalen, an institute in Big Sur, where, at the time, the most respected *yoga* teachers in North America delivered workshops. My own personal hero, Carl Jung, spent time there. All the great minds of spirituality have passed through Esalen.

Esalen is built on a rock on Native American land, overlooking the ocean. According to the Native Americans it's a magical place because water from the hot springs, the creek, and the ocean blend together on this land. The energies at Esalen are extremely powerful, and one can sense them the moment one arrives

After having taken all the main *yoga* workshops, I needed more than someone else's contemporary interpretation of *yoga*. I needed to go straight to the source—the scriptures written by the great sages and gurus that were preserving the teachings as they were taught when *yoga* initially flourished. I read all the *yogic* and *tantric* scriptures I could find that have been translated into English. My time on the grounds at Esalen led to my fascination with all of the facets of *yoga*, and I changed my career path so I could devote myself to teaching *yoga* full-time. Esalen is still my sanctuary, the ashram I'd hoped to find in India but never had the chance to find. I believe that, if you are truly intent on finding *yoga*, *yoga* will find you in one form or another.

I feel lucky I ended up in California because here, my path magically crossed with some of the direct disciples of *Patthabi Jois* and *BKS Iyengar*, the most famous disciples of *Krishnamacharya*, the father of modern *yoga*. One could say they are responsible for having brought *yoga* to the west. I also pursued my *Kriya Yoga* studies in the lineage of *Yogananda*. *Kriya Yoga* focuses on

Leila Worby

meditation, while *Ashtanga Yoga* and *Iyengar Yoga* focus more on movement meditation, coupled with breathing techniques, or *pranayama*.

I was always hungry for more, so I cultivated a long love affair with *Kundalini Yoga* and *Classical Tantric Yoga*. The experience of *yoga* wasn't enough, so I ventured into the scriptures to really understand why *yoga* made me feel whole.

I still remember when *yoga* clicked for me on an intellectual level. I was studying *yogic* philosophy when I had the profound realization that *I am not my mind*. I had often been disappointed by how shallow and primitive my mind seemed to be working most of the time. By acknowledging that the nature of the mind is petty and primitive and that I shouldn't *identify* with my mind, but with my soul or true inner essence, I felt at ease. Believing that my soul was connected to a greater soul that encompasses everything was life-changing for me.

Ultimately, *yoga* is really about uniting with that omnipresent soul. Once you start developing a relationship with your soul, or your true inner essence, it becomes this cozy, safe resting place that gives you all the love and support you previously tried to find externally. And once I found this inner bliss, I felt called to share it with others.

Teaching *yoga* has taught me so much about how people are affected by stress. When people suffer from stress for long periods of time, their defenses and ability to cope with stressful events are undermined. When that happens, even the smallest incidents can seem too stressful to cope with, because of the already heightened state of the nervous system. We are all unique in how we process trauma. Just like we can't measure someone else's physical pain, we're unable to measure the gravity of someone's emotional discord. The only thing that is certain is that life is a series of traumas. Just like the great Buddha taught us, "Life is suffering."

The only thing we have the power to do is to master and direct our own mind. And this is where *yoga* and the techniques I have outlined in this book can have a tremendous impact. If we focus on the light, we can become light, and if we focus on the darkness, we can become darkness.

It's good to choose wisely.

ACKNOWLEDGEMENTS

I've never had a sole Guru, but on my path I have met many light-bearers who have profoundly touched me and inspired my practice. It's only right to mention some of them and how they illuminated me, so, if you are inclined, you can continue your studies with them.

Shanti Rubenstone at the *Yogananda Church of Self Realization* in Palo Alto

Shanti, or any Church of Self Realization, are great resources if you wish to explore *Kriya Yoga*.

Beata Skrzypacz

If you want to study in the *Ashtanga Yoga* lineage, Beata is my teacher of choice. She has a very balanced, non-dogmatic view of the practice.

Kirsten Berg and Mitchell Gold

Direct disciples of Pattabhi Jois, this couple have illuminated the core teachings of *Ashtanga Yoga* to me, beyond just the poses. If you're ever in Bali and want to study one of the root traditions of *Yoga* I recommend seeking out this duo.

Christopher Wallis

Christopher Wallis has translated some of the core scriptures of *Classical Nondual Shaiva Tantra* to English, and I recommend reading his book: *Tantra Illuminated*. If you are cerebrally oriented and thirst for a deeper understanding and integration of the scriptures, I recommend studying with Christopher.

Shiva Rea

Shiva's style of *yoga* is called *Prana Vinyasa and allows* you to move like the elements. Her gift to the *yoga* community is a complete embodied experience of *tantra*. If you are burned out on traditional *yoga* or just want a practice that feels exquisite, seek this woman out.

Sally Kempton

Sally is a good resource if you are getting more acquainted with the *kundalini* energy. If you are interested in deepening your meditation and you want to experience it from a *tantric* perspective, seek this woman out.

Ananda Yogiji and Jaya Lakshmi

If you are interested in exploring the path of devotion (*Bhakti Yoga)*, through chanting, I would recommend seeking this duo out. They are talented musicians and I recommend exploring some of their recordings.

Kia Miller

If you're interested in exploring *Kundalini Yoga* and the energy body, seek this teacher out. She is well versed in many lineages of *Classical Yoga*.

INDEX

Made in the USA
Las Vegas, NV
10 October 2023